BEGINNERS DELICIOUS HIGH-PROTEIN DIET RECIPES

ANUSHA A

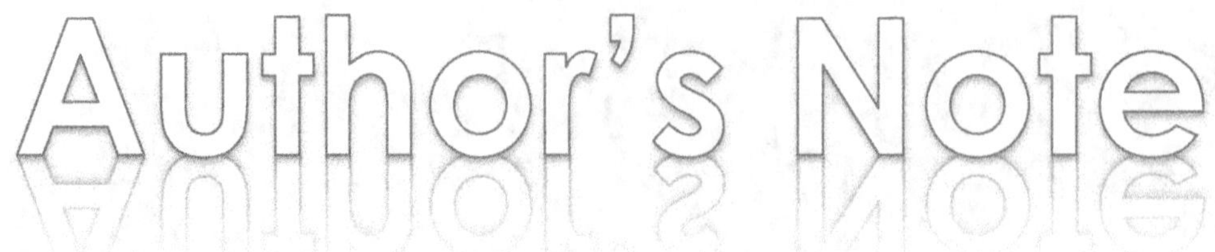

Author's Note

Dear Readers

THERE IS LOT TO EXPERIENCE IN LIFETIME – START EXPLORE!!

As you embark on your path to success, keep in mind that you have the ability to attain your goals and desires. You will have challenges and setbacks along the way, but it is critical that you remain resilient and keep going forward. Each difficulty provides an opportunity for growth and learning, and each step puts you closer to your objectives. Be confident in yourself and your ability. You are capable of great things, and your distinct abilities and characteristics have the ability to positively impact the world around you. Accept your full potential and dare to dream large. Find inspiration in the stories of people who overcame adversity and succeeded despite the odds. Their stories serve as reminders that with determination, perseverance, and hard work, anything is possible. Surround yourself with happiness and encouragement. Seek for mentors, friends, and colleagues who can encourage and motivate you on your journey. Their advice, wisdom, and support can give you the inspiration you need to keep going, even when things get rough. Remember to acknowledge your progress and accomplishments along the way, no matter how minor they may appear. Each achievement is a credit to your hard work and commitment. Above all, trust in the journey and have faith in yourself. Believe that you are deserving of success and that your efforts will be rewarded in due time. Keep striving, keep believing, and never lose sight of the vision you have for your life. You are capable, you are resilient, and you are destined for greatness. Let your journey be guided by courage, optimism, and a relentless pursuit of your dreams. The world is waiting for you to shine your light brightly and make your mark. Keep going, keep growing, and never lose sight of the incredible potential that lies within you.

With warmest wishes for your success.

[Ms. Anusha]

*Some pictures are downloaded from META AI for the illustration purpose there is no intend to steal any one works pictures used here are to explain how the output will turn at end.

Introduction

A high-protein diet is becoming more popular among fitness enthusiasts, athletes, and anyone trying to improve their overall health and wellness.

This diet concentrates on protein-rich foods that aid in muscle growth and repair, induce satiety, and support metabolic activities.

Protein is one of three macronutrients required for physical activities, along with carbohydrates and fats, but it has the distinct advantage of being extremely effective for muscle growth and weight management.

The Importance of Protein

Protein is essential for tissue maintenance and repair, enzyme and hormone production, and muscle development. When you consume protein,

your body converts it into amino acids, which are then employed in a variety of biological processes. A high-protein diet can be especially useful for those

who live an active lifestyle or want to reduce weight because protein helps to sustain lean muscle mass while also increasing fat loss.

Furthermore, protein has a thermogenic impact, which means your body expends more energy to breakdown it than fats or carbohydrates. This can lead to more calorie burning and a faster metabolism.

Protein-rich meals also help you feel fuller for longer, which reduces cravings and prevents overeating.

Who Benefits From a High-Protein Diet?

A high-protein diet is adaptable and may be tailored to a variety of health and fitness objectives. Athletes and bodybuilders frequently rely on protein to aid in muscle repair and growth following strenuous exercise.

Protein is important for weight loss because it helps maintain muscle mass, which burns more calories than fat even at rest. Furthermore, those with certain medical disorders,

such as type 2 diabetes, may benefit from increased protein intake since it helps regulate blood sugar levels and promotes a healthy body weight.

It is crucial to understand that not all proteins are created equal. Complete proteins, which include all nine essential amino acids, are commonly found in animal products such as meat, fish, eggs, and dairy.

Plant-based dieters can still reap the benefits of a high-protein diet by combining foods such as beans, lentils, quinoa, and tofu to achieve a complete amino acid profile.

High Protein Diet Recipes: What to Expect

When following a high-protein diet, diversity is essential for keeping meals enjoyable and nutritionally balanced. This collection of high-protein recipes contains options for every meal—breakfast, lunch,

supper, and even snacks—allowing you to eat tasty food while reaching your protein objectives. Whether you're looking for hefty meat dishes, satisfying vegetarian options, or quick protein-packed snacks, you'll find lots of ideas here.

Expect recipes that are high in protein, vitamins, minerals, and healthy fats. There's something for every taste and dietary inclination, from traditional

grilled chicken recipes to more innovative options such as protein-packed smoothies and baked pastries created with protein powder.

Tips for Succeed on a High Protein Diet

To reap the full advantages of a high-protein diet, aim for a variety of protein sources and don't overlook other macronutrients such as healthy fats and complex carbohydrates.

Stay hydrated, as your body need extra water to absorb protein, and consider speaking with a nutritionist to verify you're fulfilling your unique nutritional requirements.

Also, make sure to include both animal and plant-based proteins for a well-rounded approach, ensuring that your meals are nutrient-dense and sustainable over time.

By focusing on nutrient-dense, high-protein meals, you'll be well on your way to meeting your health and fitness objectives.

Table of Content

13. Keto BLT Salad

14. Garlic Lemon Butter Scallops

15. Cauliflower Fried Rice

16. Keto Cloud Bread

17. Bacon-Wrapped Asparagus

18. Keto Chicken Tacos (Lettuce Wraps)

19. Keto Cheeseburger Casserole

20. Broccoli and Cheddar Soup

21. Quinoa Salad with Chickpeas and Feta

22. Sweet Potato anELEGENT ART OF CHICKEN COOKERY

23. Spaghetti Bolognese

24. Pasta Primavera

25. Chicken Pita Wraps

26. Oven-Roasted Potatoes and Brussels Sprouts

27. Stuffed Bell Peppers

28. Vegetable Risotto

29. Whole Wheat Veggie Pizza

30. Mediterranean Couscous Salad

31. Butternut Squash Soup

32. Whole Wheat Pita Bread with Hummus

33. Chickpea and Spinach Stew

34. Stuffed Zucchini Boats

35. Oatmeal with Berries

36. Vegetarian Chili

37. Bulgur Wheat Tabbouleh

38. Baked Falafel Wraps

39. Mushroom and Spinach Risotto

40. Lentil and Sweet Potato Curry

41. Grilled Veggie Skewers

42. Caprese Salad

43. Eggplant Parmesan

44. Vegetable Stir Fry

45. Margherita Pizza

46. Greek Salad

47. Stuffed Grape Leaves

48. Tomato and Basil Bruschetta

49. Spinach and Feta Stuffed Peppers

50. Roasted Cauliflower Steaks

1.Keto Avocado Bacon Salad Recipe

Packed with healthy fats from avocado and bacon, this salad promotes heart health, aids in weight loss, and keeps you satisfied.

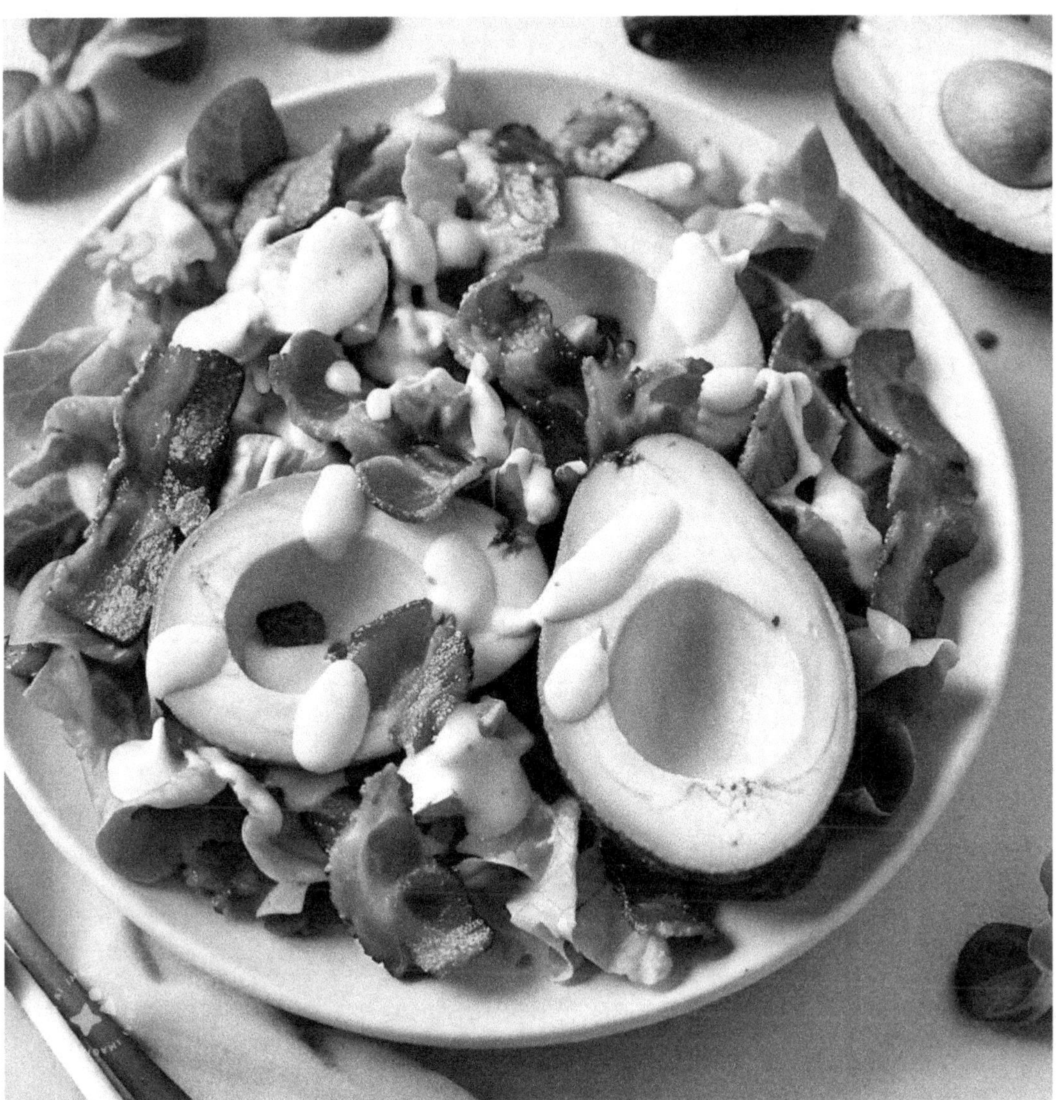

Ingredients:

- 2 ripe avocados, peeled, pitted, and diced

- 6 slices of bacon, cooked and crumbled

- 4 cups of romaine lettuce, chopped

- 1 medium cucumber, diced

- 2 tablespoons olive oil

- 1 tablespoon lime juice (freshly squeezed)

- Salt and pepper, to taste

- Optional: ¼ cup red onion, thinly sliced

Instructions:

1. Prepare the bacon:

  - Cook the bacon in a skillet over medium heat until crispy. Remove from the pan, place it on a paper towel to drain the excess fat, and crumble it into bite-sized pieces. Set aside.

2. Chop the vegetables:

  - While the bacon is cooking, chop the romaine lettuce, dice the cucumber, and slice the avocados. You can also thinly slice the red onion if you are using it.

3. Make the dressing:

  - In a small bowl, whisk together the olive oil, lime juice, salt, and pepper. Adjust seasoning to your preference.

4. Assemble the salad:

  - In a large bowl, combine the chopped romaine lettuce, diced avocado, cucumber, and crumbled bacon. If using, add the red onion slices.

5. Dress the salad:

  - Drizzle the olive oil and lime dressing over the salad and gently toss to combine, ensuring the ingredients are evenly coated.

6. Serve immediately:

  - Enjoy your fresh Keto Avocado Bacon Salad as a light lunch or a healthy side dish!

2. Garlic Butter Shrimp Zoodles Recipe

Zoodles provide a low-carb alternative to pasta, while shrimp provide a lean protein source high in omega-3s and antioxidants.

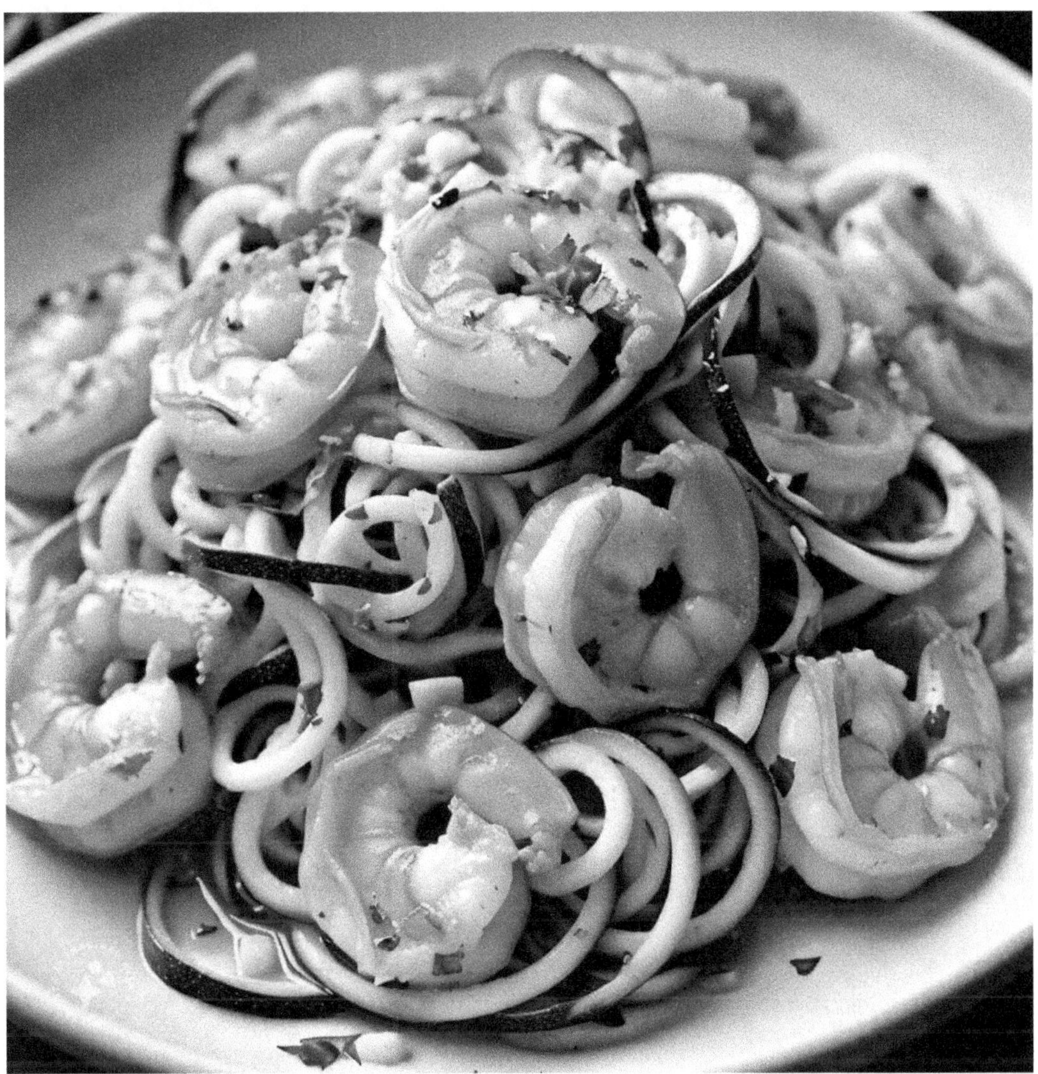

Ingredients:

- 1 lb (450g) shrimp, peeled and deveined

- 3 medium zucchini, spiralized into noodles (zoodles)

- 3 tablespoons unsalted butter

- 4 garlic cloves, minced

- 1 tablespoon olive oil

- 1 tablespoon lemon juice (freshly squeezed)

- Salt and pepper, to taste

- ¼ teaspoon red pepper flakes (optional)

- 2 tablespoons fresh parsley, chopped (for garnish)

- Optional: grated Parmesan cheese for serving

Instructions:

1. Prepare the zoodles:

   - Spiralize the zucchini into noodles using a spiralizer or a vegetable peeler. Set the zoodles aside while you prepare the shrimp.

2. Cook the shrimp:

   - In a large skillet, heat the olive oil and 1 tablespoon of butter over medium heat.

   - Add the minced garlic and sauté for 1 minute until fragrant, but not browned.

   - Add the shrimp to the skillet, season with salt, pepper, and red pepper flakes (if using). Cook the shrimp for about 2-3 minutes on each side, or until they turn pink and opaque.

   - Once cooked, remove the shrimp from the skillet and set aside.

3. Make the garlic butter sauce:

   - In the same skillet, add the remaining 2 tablespoons of butter. Once melted, add the lemon juice and stir to combine. Let the sauce simmer for about 1-2 minutes.

4. Cook the zoodles:

   - Add the spiralized zucchini noodles (zoodles) to the skillet with the garlic butter sauce. Cook for about 2-3 minutes, tossing gently until the zoodles are tender but still have a slight crunch (al dente). Do not overcook, as they will become soggy.

5. Combine shrimp and zoodles:

   - Return the cooked shrimp to the skillet and toss with the zoodles, ensuring everything is well coated in the garlic butter sauce.

6. Serve:

   - Garnish with chopped fresh parsley and, if desired, sprinkle some grated Parmesan cheese on top. Serve immediately.

3. Keto Cauliflower Mac and Cheese Recipe

Cauliflower is a nutrient-dense, low-carb alternative to pasta, whilst cheese contains necessary fats and protein.

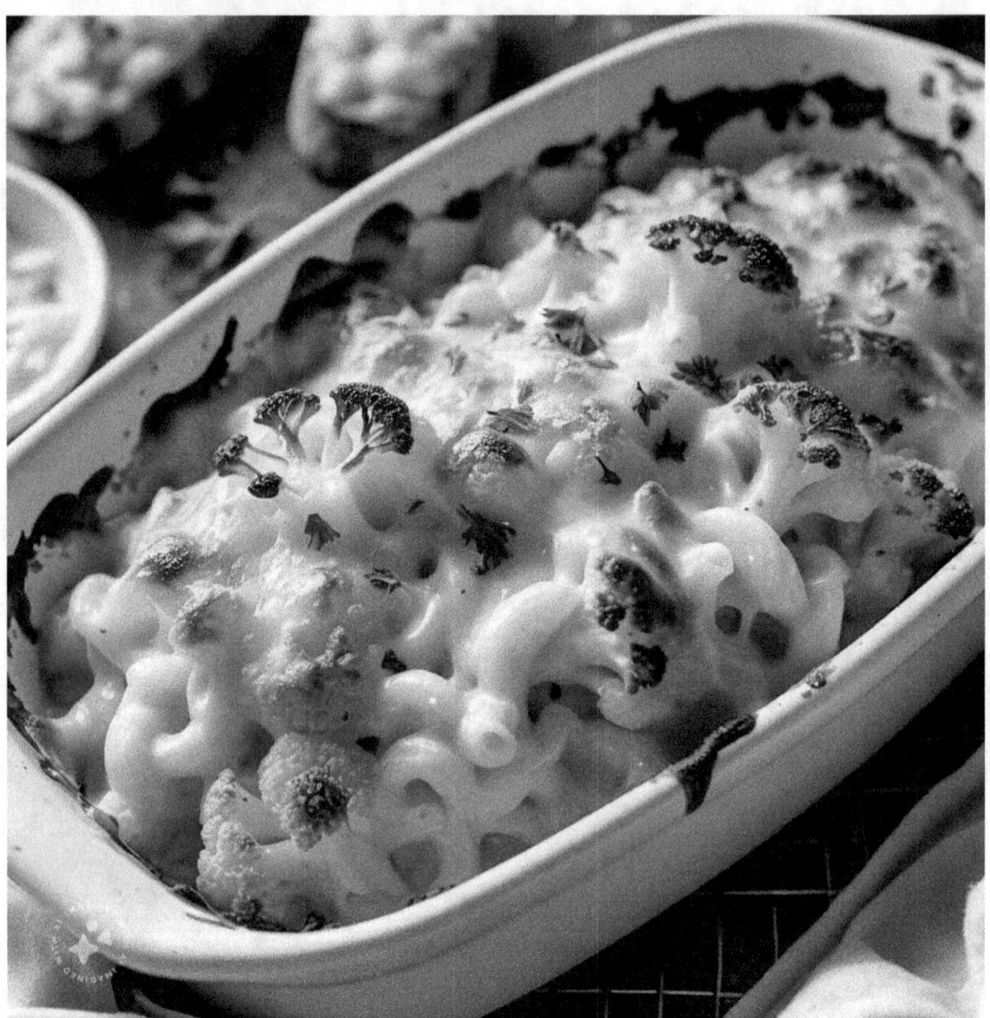

Ingredients:

- 1 large head of cauliflower, cut into florets

- 1 ½ cups shredded cheddar cheese

- 4 oz cream cheese, softened

- ½ cup heavy cream

- ¼ cup grated Parmesan cheese

- 2 tablespoons butter

- 1 teaspoon garlic powder

- ½ teaspoon onion powder

- Salt and pepper, to taste

- Optional: ¼ teaspoon paprika or cayenne pepper for added spice

- Optional: ¼ cup pork rinds, crushed

Instructions:

1. Preheat the oven:

  - Preheat your oven to 375°F (190°C) and grease a medium-sized baking dish.

2. Prepare the cauliflower:

  - Bring a large pot of salted water to a boil. Add the cauliflower florets and cook for about 5-7 minutes, or until the cauliflower is tender but still firm (al dente). Drain well and pat the cauliflower dry with a paper towel to remove excess moisture.

3. Make the cheese sauce:

  - In a large saucepan, melt the butter over medium heat. Add the cream cheese and stir until it melts and becomes smooth.

  - Gradually stir in the heavy cream and continue cooking for 2-3 minutes until the mixture is fully combined.

  - Add the shredded cheddar cheese and Parmesan cheese, stirring until the cheeses melt and the sauce becomes thick and creamy. Season with garlic powder, onion powder, salt, and pepper. For added spice, stir in paprika or cayenne pepper if desired.

4. Assemble the mac and cheese:

  - Add the cooked cauliflower florets to the cheese sauce and stir until the cauliflower is fully coated with the sauce.

5. Bake:

  - Transfer the cauliflower and cheese mixture to the prepared baking dish. If you'd like a crispy topping, sprinkle the crushed pork rinds over the top.

  - Bake in the preheated oven for 15-20 minutes, or until the top is golden brown and the cheese is bubbly.

6. Serve:

  - Remove from the oven and let it cool for a few minutes before serving. Enjoy your keto-friendly cauliflower mac and cheese!

4. Crispy Keto Chicken Wings Recipe

Chicken wings are high in protein and low in carbohydrates, providing a delicious crunch without disrupting ketosis.

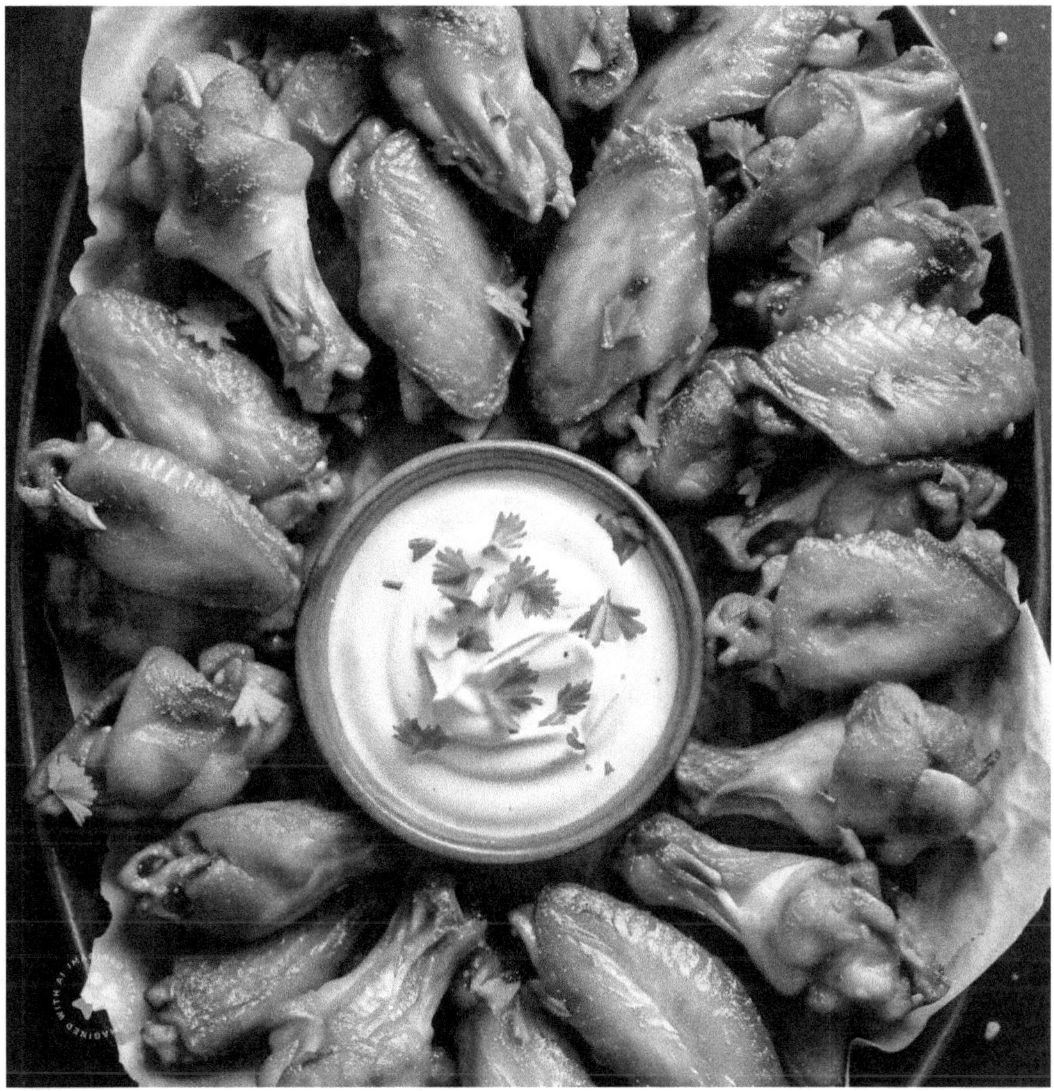

Ingredients:

- 2 lbs (900g) chicken wings, split into flats and drumettes

- 2 tablespoons baking powder (aluminum-free)

- 1 teaspoon garlic powder

- 1 teaspoon onion powder

- 1 teaspoon paprika

- ½ teaspoon salt

- ½ teaspoon black pepper

- ½ cup buffalo sauce (store-bought or homemade)

- 2 tablespoons unsalted butter (melted)

- Optional: 1 tablespoon chopped fresh parsley (for garnish)

Instructions:

1. Preheat the oven:

  - Preheat your oven to 400°F (200°C) and line a large baking sheet with foil. Place a wire rack on top of the baking sheet to elevate the wings for better crisping.

2. Prepare the wings:

  - Pat the chicken wings dry with paper towels to remove excess moisture. This step is important for achieving crispy skin.

3. Coat the wings:

  - In a large bowl, mix the baking powder, garlic powder, onion powder, paprika, salt, and black pepper.

  - Toss the chicken wings in the seasoning mixture until they are evenly coated. The baking powder will help the wings become extra crispy as they bake.

4. Bake the wings:

  - Place the seasoned wings on the wire rack, ensuring they are spaced out so the air can circulate around them.

  - Bake in the preheated oven for 40-45 minutes, flipping halfway through, until the wings are golden brown and crispy.

5. Make the buffalo sauce:

- While the wings are baking, melt the butter in a small saucepan or microwave.

- In a separate bowl, mix the melted butter with the buffalo sauce until well combined.

6. Toss the wings in sauce:

- Once the wings are fully cooked and crispy, remove them from the oven. Toss the hot wings in the buffalo sauce mixture, ensuring they are well coated.

7. Serve:

- Garnish with chopped fresh parsley (optional) and serve immediately with your favorite keto-friendly dipping sauce, such as ranch or blue cheese dressing.

5.Zucchini Lasagna Recipe

Zucchini slices minimize carbs, while layers of cheese and meat add protein and necessary lipids.

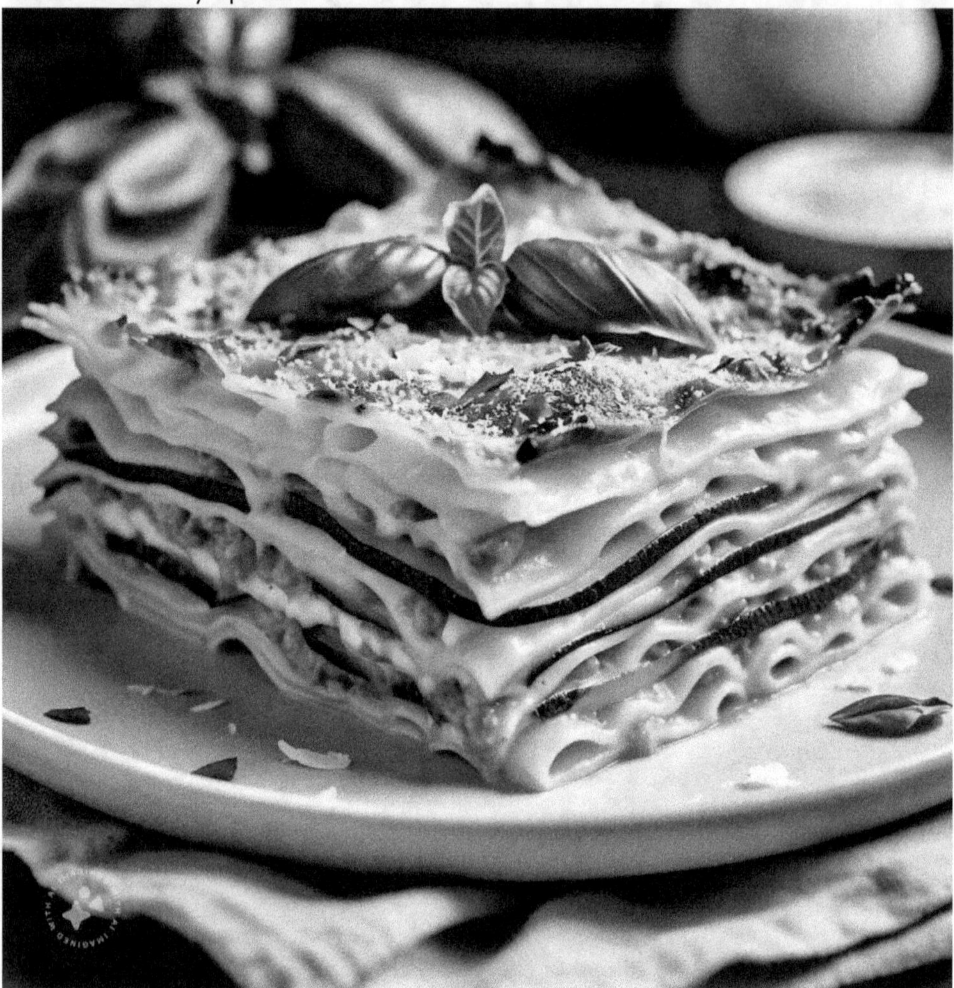

Ingredients:

- 3 large zucchinis, thinly sliced lengthwise

- 1 lb (450g) ground beef (or ground turkey)

- 1 cup ricotta cheese

- 1 ½ cups shredded mozzarella cheese

- 1 cup grated Parmesan cheese

- 2 cups marinara sauce

- 1 egg

- 2 cloves garlic, minced

- 1 small onion, finely chopped

- 1 tablespoon olive oil

- 1 teaspoon Italian seasoning

- ½ teaspoon salt

- ½ teaspoon black pepper

- Fresh basil or parsley (optional for garnish)

Instructions:

1. Preheat the oven:

   - Preheat your oven to 375°F (190°C) and grease a 9x13-inch baking dish.

2. Prepare the zucchini slices:

   - Using a mandoline or a sharp knife, thinly slice the zucchinis lengthwise into ⅛-inch thick slices.

   - Lay the zucchini slices on paper towels, sprinkle lightly with salt, and let them sit for 10-15 minutes to draw out moisture. Afterward, pat them dry with another paper towel. This step prevents the lasagna from becoming watery.

3. Cook the beef filling:

   - In a large skillet, heat the olive oil over medium heat. Add the chopped onion and minced garlic, cooking until softened (about 2-3 minutes).

   - Add the ground beef, Italian seasoning, salt, and pepper, and cook until the beef is browned and fully cooked (about 7-8 minutes). Drain any excess fat.

   - Stir in the marinara sauce and let the mixture simmer for 5 minutes. Remove from heat and set aside.

4. Prepare the ricotta mixture:

   - In a medium bowl, mix the ricotta cheese, egg, ½ cup of the Parmesan cheese, and a pinch of salt and pepper. Set aside.

5. Assemble the lasagna:

- Spread a thin layer of the meat sauce at the bottom of the greased baking dish.

- Lay a layer of zucchini slices on top of the sauce, followed by half of the ricotta mixture.

- Add a layer of the meat sauce on top of the ricotta, followed by a sprinkle of shredded mozzarella and Parmesan.

- Repeat the layers, starting with zucchini, until all ingredients are used. Finish with a top layer of meat sauce and a generous amount of shredded mozzarella and Parmesan.

6. Bake:

- Cover the baking dish with foil and bake in the preheated oven for 30 minutes.

- Remove the foil and bake for an additional 15-20 minutes until the cheese is bubbly and golden brown.

7. Let it rest:

- Once baked, allow the zucchini lasagna to rest for 10-15 minutes before slicing and serving. This helps the layers set and makes it easier to cut.

8. Serve:

- Garnish with fresh basil or parsley if desired and enjoy your keto-friendly zucchini lasagna!

6. Keto Salmon with Avocado Salsa Recipe

Salmon's omega-3s, combined with avocado's monounsaturated fats, have anti-inflammatory properties.

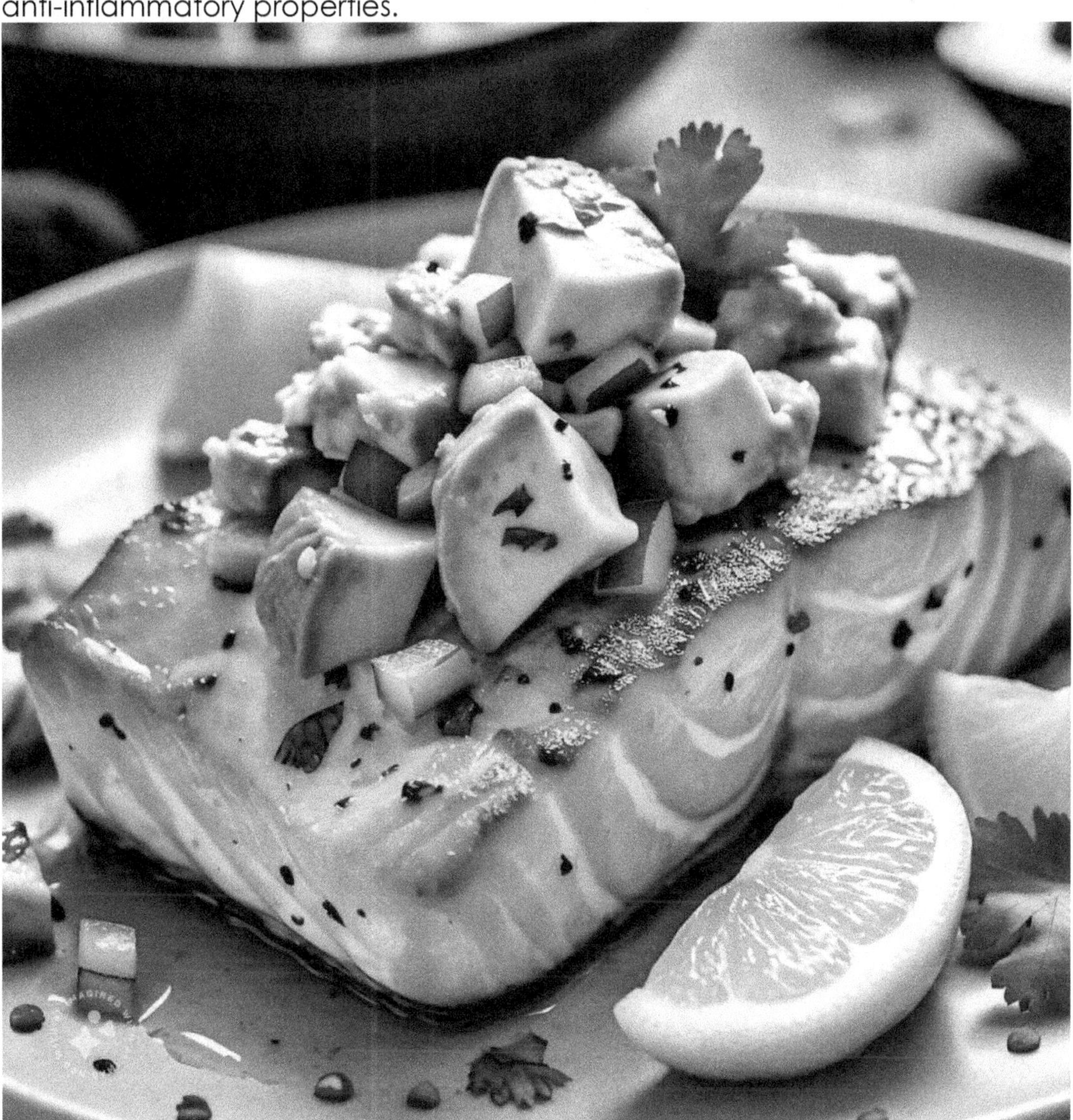

Ingredients:

For the Salmon:

- 4 salmon fillets (about 6 oz each)

- 2 tablespoons olive oil

- 1 teaspoon garlic powder

- 1 teaspoon paprika

- ½ teaspoon ground cumin

- ½ teaspoon salt

- ½ teaspoon black pepper

- 1 tablespoon fresh lemon juice

For the Avocado Salsa:

- 2 ripe avocados, diced

- 1 medium tomato, diced

- ¼ cup red onion, finely chopped

- 2 tablespoons fresh cilantro, chopped

- 1 tablespoon olive oil

- 1 tablespoon lime juice (freshly squeezed)

- Salt and pepper, to taste

Instructions:

1. Prepare the salmon:

  - In a small bowl, mix the olive oil, garlic powder, paprika, cumin, salt, pepper, and lemon juice.

  - Brush this mixture over the salmon fillets, ensuring they are evenly coated. Let the salmon sit for 10-15 minutes to marinate.

2. Make the avocado salsa:

  - In a medium bowl, combine the diced avocados, tomato, red onion, and cilantro.

  - Drizzle with olive oil and lime juice, and season with salt and pepper. Gently toss the ingredients together until well combined. Set the salsa aside while you cook the salmon.

3. Grill the salmon:

  - Preheat a grill or stovetop grill pan over medium-high heat. Lightly oil the grates to prevent sticking.

- Place the salmon fillets on the grill, skin-side down, and cook for 4-5 minutes per side, or until the salmon is fully cooked through and flakes easily with a fork. Adjust the cooking time based on the thickness of the fillets.

4. Serve:

- Once the salmon is cooked, transfer the fillets to plates and top each one with a generous portion of the avocado salsa.

- Serve immediately, garnished with extra lime wedges or cilantro if desired.

7.Spinach and Cheese Stuffed Mushrooms

This low-carb, nutrient-dense recipe combines mushrooms and spinach, both of which are rich in antioxidants.

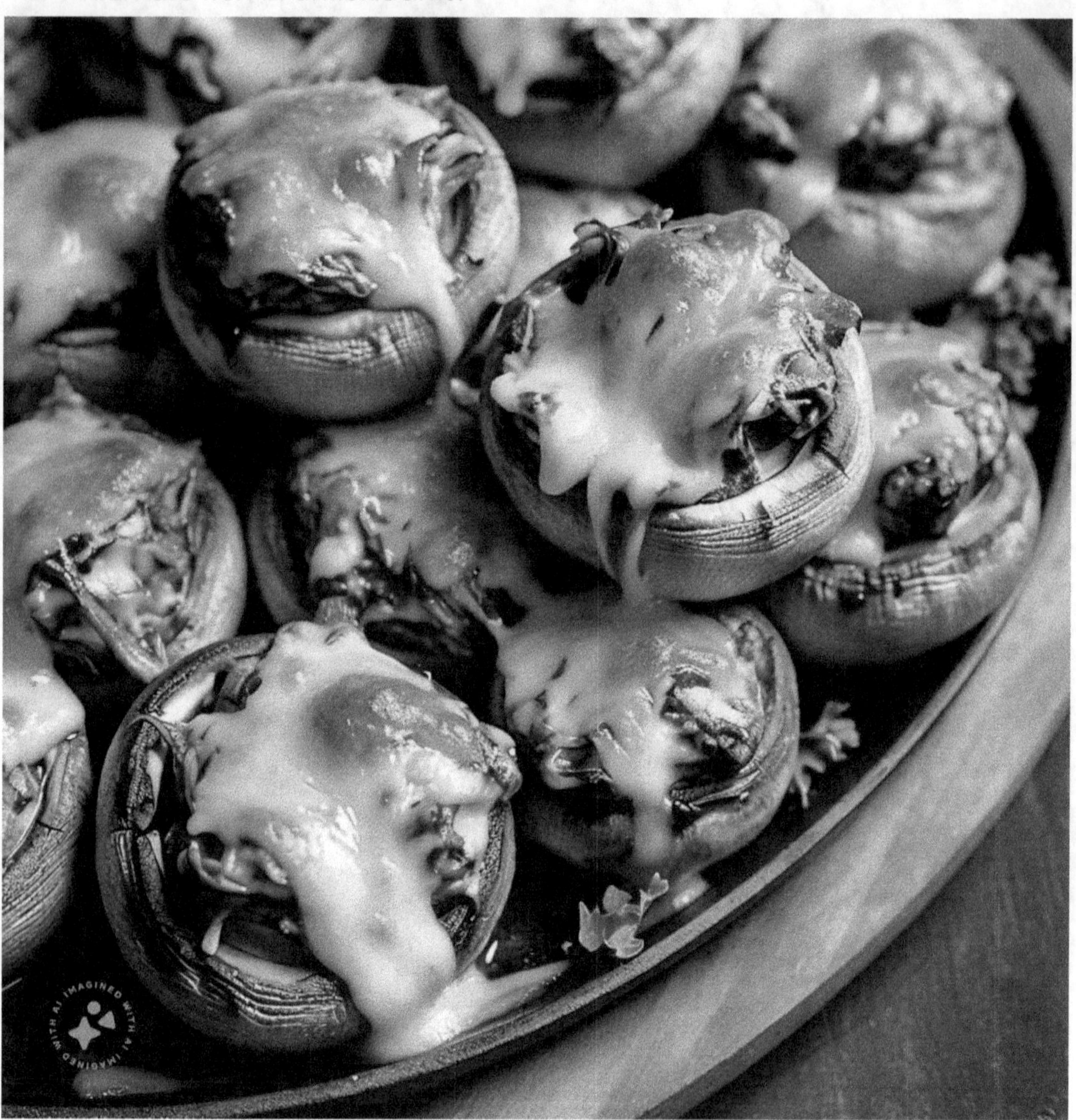

Ingredients:

- 20 large button mushrooms, stems removed and cleaned

- 2 cups fresh spinach, chopped

- 1/2 cup cream cheese, softened

- 1/4 cup grated Parmesan cheese

- 2 cloves garlic, minced

- 1 tablespoon olive oil

- 1/4 teaspoon salt

- 1/4 teaspoon black pepper

- 1/4 teaspoon red pepper flakes (optional)

- 2 tablespoons breadcrumbs (optional for added crunch)

- Fresh parsley, chopped (for garnish)

Instructions:

1. **Prepare the Mushrooms:**

   - Preheat your oven to 190°C (375°F). Line a baking sheet with parchment paper or lightly grease it with oil.

   - Clean the mushrooms thoroughly, removing the stems and gently scraping out the inside if needed to create more room for the filling.

2. **Cook the Spinach:**

   - Heat the olive oil in a pan over medium heat. Add the minced garlic and cook until fragrant, about 1 minute.

   - Add the chopped spinach to the pan and cook for 3-4 minutes until wilted. Remove from heat and let it cool slightly.

3. **Prepare the Filling:**

   - In a mixing bowl, combine the cooked spinach, cream cheese, Parmesan, salt, black pepper, and red pepper flakes (if using).

   - Mix everything together until well combined.

4. **Stuff the Mushrooms:**

   - Using a small spoon, carefully fill each mushroom cap with the spinach and cheese mixture. If desired, sprinkle the top of each stuffed mushroom with breadcrumbs for extra texture.

5. **Bake:**

   - Place the stuffed mushrooms on the prepared baking sheet and bake in the preheated oven for 20-25 minutes or until the mushrooms are tender and the tops are golden brown.

6. **Garnish and Serve:**

   - Once baked, remove the mushrooms from the oven and sprinkle with freshly chopped parsley for garnish.

   - Serve warm as an appetizer or side dish.

8. Keto Beef and Broccoli Stir Fry

Packed with protein and fiber, this low-carb stir fry regulates blood sugar levels and promotes metabolism.

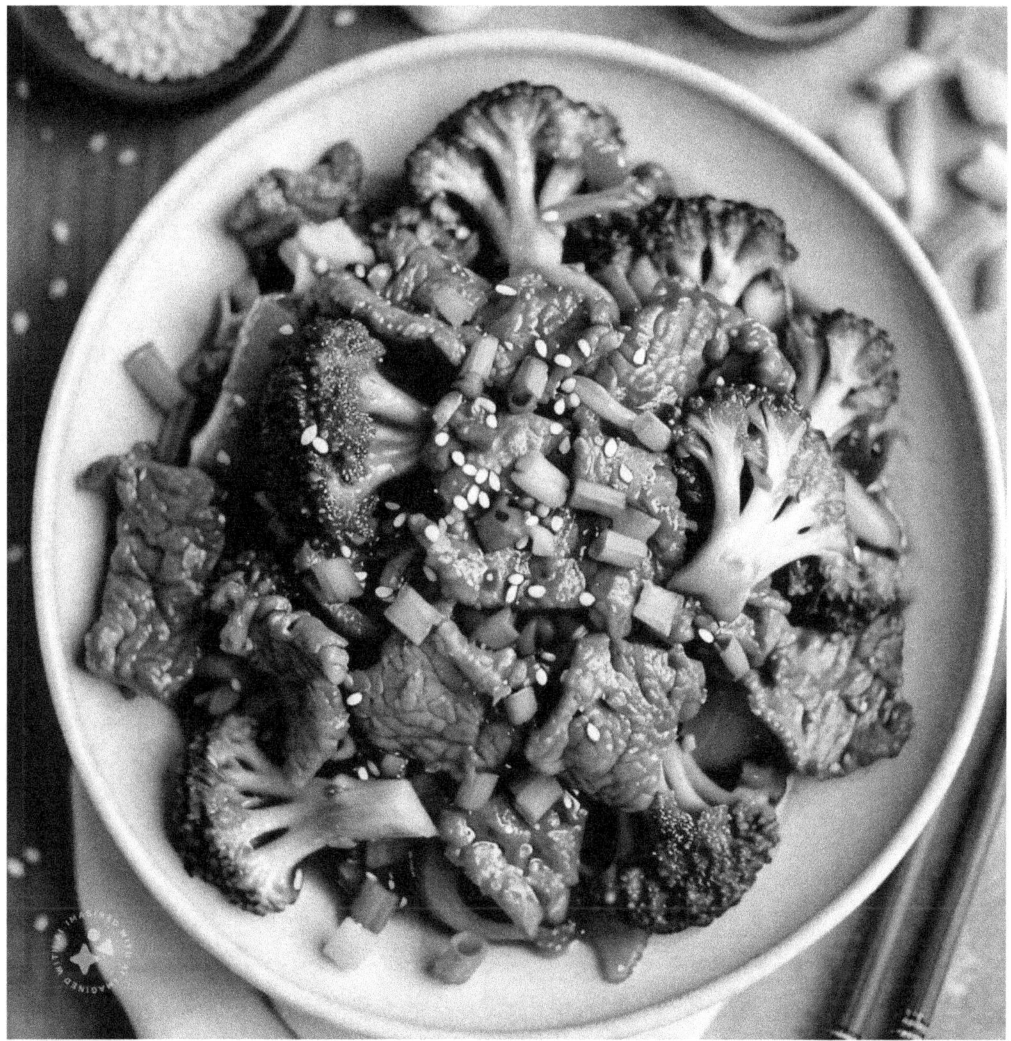

Ingredients:

- 450g (1 lb) beef sirloin or flank steak, thinly sliced

- 3 cups broccoli florets

- 2 tablespoons soy sauce (or tamari for gluten-free)

- 2 tablespoons sesame oil

- 2 tablespoons olive oil (or avocado oil)

- 2 cloves garlic, minced

- 1 tablespoon fresh ginger, minced

- 1 tablespoon rice vinegar

- 1 tablespoon sesame seeds

- 1/2 teaspoon red pepper flakes (optional)

- Salt and pepper, to taste

- Sliced green onions (for garnish)

Instructions:

1. **Prepare the Beef:**

   - Thinly slice the beef into bite-sized strips. Season with salt and pepper.

2. **Blanch the Broccoli:**

   - Bring a pot of water to a boil and add the broccoli florets. Blanch for about 2 minutes until bright green and tender but still crisp.

   - Drain and set aside.

3. **Cook the Beef:**

   - Heat 1 tablespoon of olive oil in a large pan or wok over medium-high heat.

   - Add the beef slices in batches (to avoid overcrowding) and stir-fry for 2-3 minutes until browned and cooked through.

   - Remove the beef from the pan and set aside.

4. **Stir-fry the Aromatics:**

   - In the same pan, add the remaining 1 tablespoon of olive oil. Add the minced garlic and ginger, and cook for 1-2 minutes until fragrant.

5. **Combine Ingredients:**

   - Return the cooked beef to the pan along with the blanched broccoli.

   - Pour in the soy sauce, sesame oil, rice vinegar, and red pepper flakes (if using). Stir everything together and cook for another 2-3 minutes, allowing the sauce to coat the beef and broccoli.

6. **Serve:**

   - Garnish with sesame seeds and sliced green onions, and serve hot.

9.Keto Egg Muffins

These egg muffins provide a quick, protein-packed breakfast that promotes muscle maintenance and energy.

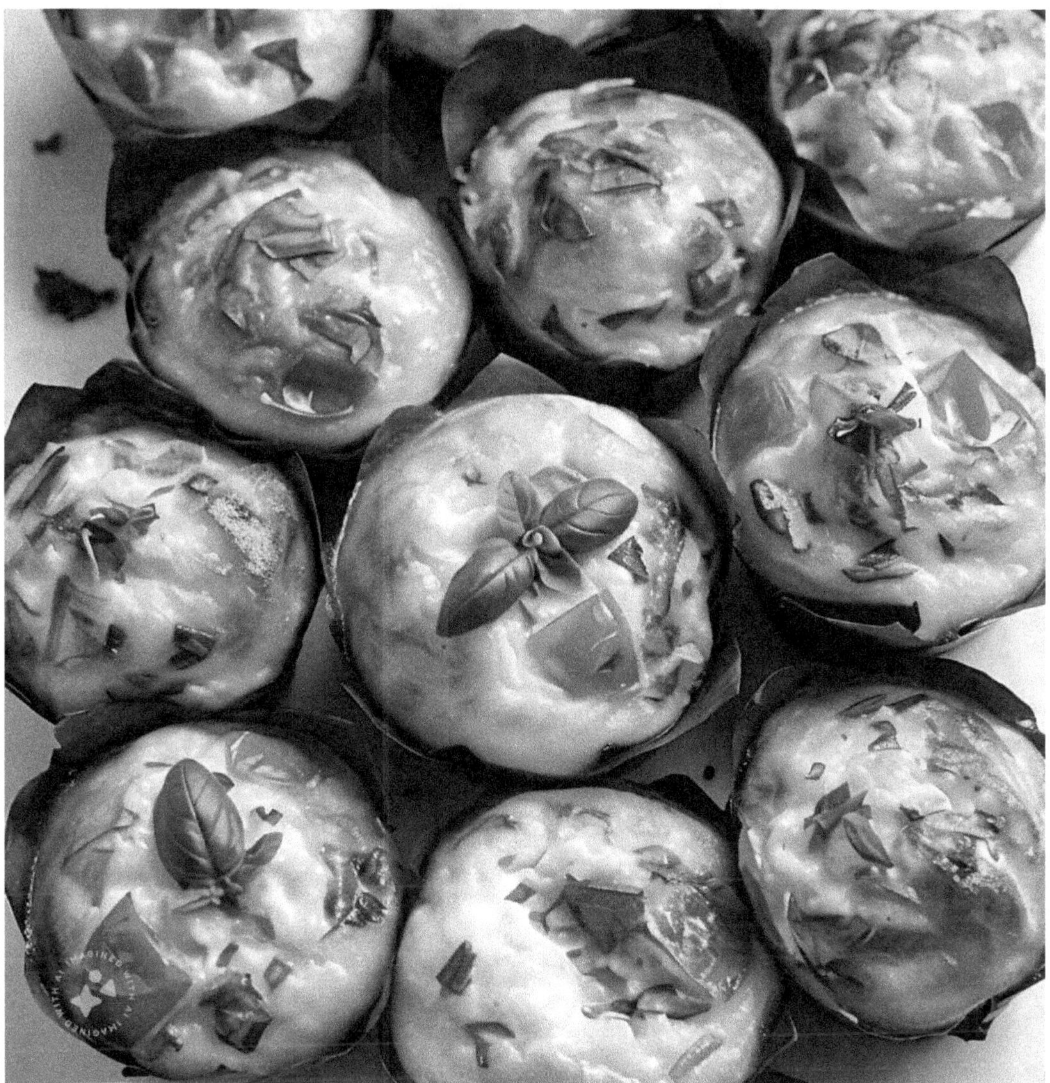

Ingredients:

- 6 large eggs

- 1/2 cup spinach, chopped

- 1/2 cup shredded cheese (cheddar, mozzarella, or your choice)

- 4 slices bacon, cooked and crumbled

- 1/4 cup heavy cream (optional for creaminess)

- 1/4 teaspoon salt

- 1/4 teaspoon black pepper

- 1/4 teaspoon garlic powder (optional)

- 1/4 teaspoon paprika (optional)

- Non-stick cooking spray or oil for greasing the muffin tin

Instructions:

1. **Preheat the Oven:**

   - Preheat your oven to 180°C (350°F). Lightly grease a 6-cup muffin tin with cooking spray or oil.

2. **Prepare the Egg Mixture:**

   - In a medium-sized mixing bowl, crack the eggs and whisk them until smooth.

   - Add the heavy cream (if using), salt, black pepper, garlic powder, and paprika. Whisk until everything is combined.

3. **Add the Fillings:**

   - Stir in the chopped spinach, shredded cheese, and crumbled bacon into the egg mixture, making sure the ingredients are evenly distributed.

4. **Fill the Muffin Cups:**

   - Pour the egg mixture into the prepared muffin tin, filling each cup about 3/4 full to allow room for the muffins to puff up as they bake.

5. **Bake:**

   - Place the muffin tin in the preheated oven and bake for 15-20 minutes, or until the egg muffins are set and slightly golden on top.

6. **Cool and Serve:**

   - Once baked, let the egg muffins cool in the tin for a few minutes before removing them. Serve warm.

10. Keto Chicken Alfredo

A creamy, comforting dish that combines low-carb noodles with substantial fats from cheese and chicken for a well-rounded lunch.

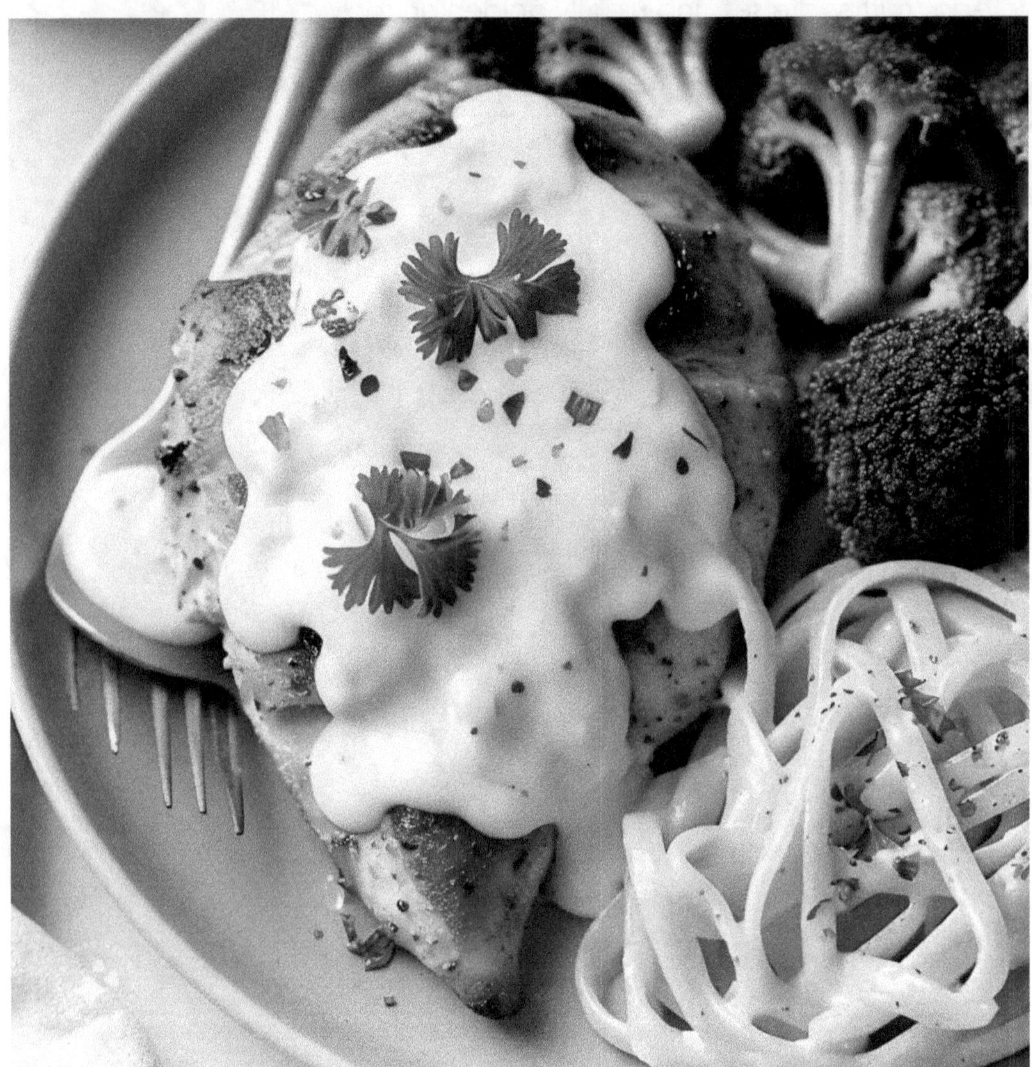

Ingredients:

- 2 medium chicken breasts, boneless and skinless

- 2 medium zucchinis, spiralized into noodles (zoodles)

- 1 tablespoon olive oil

- Salt and pepper, to taste

For the Alfredo Sauce:

- 1 cup heavy cream

- 1/2 cup Parmesan cheese, grated

- 2 tablespoons unsalted butter

- 2 cloves garlic, minced

- 1/4 teaspoon garlic powder (optional)

- 1/4 teaspoon black pepper

- 1/4 teaspoon salt

- Fresh parsley, chopped (for garnish)

Instructions:

1. **Prepare the Chicken:**

   - Season the chicken breasts with salt and pepper on both sides.

   - Heat olive oil in a grill pan or regular skillet over medium heat.

   - Grill the chicken breasts for 6-8 minutes on each side, or until fully cooked and golden brown. Set aside and let them rest for a few minutes, then slice.

2. **Make the Alfredo Sauce:**

   - In a medium saucepan, melt the butter over medium heat.

   - Add the minced garlic and sauté for about 1 minute until fragrant.

   - Pour in the heavy cream, stirring frequently. Let the cream simmer for 3-4 minutes.

   - Stir in the Parmesan cheese, garlic powder, salt, and black pepper. Continue stirring until the sauce thickens, about 2-3 more minutes.

   - Remove from heat once the sauce reaches the desired consistency.

3. **Cook the Zucchini Noodles:**

   - While the sauce is cooking, heat a separate pan over medium heat and add a small amount of oil or butter.

   - Add the zucchini noodles and sauté for 2-3 minutes, just until they begin to soften. Be careful not to overcook them as they can become soggy.

4. **Assemble the Dish:**

   - Divide the zucchini noodles into serving plates. Top with the grilled chicken slices.

   - Pour the Alfredo sauce generously over the chicken and zoodles.

5. **Garnish and Serve:**

   - Garnish with freshly chopped parsley and more Parmesan if desired. Serve immediately.

11. Coconut Flour Pancakes

These pancakes are high in fiber but low in carbs, which aids digestion and reduces sugar cravings.

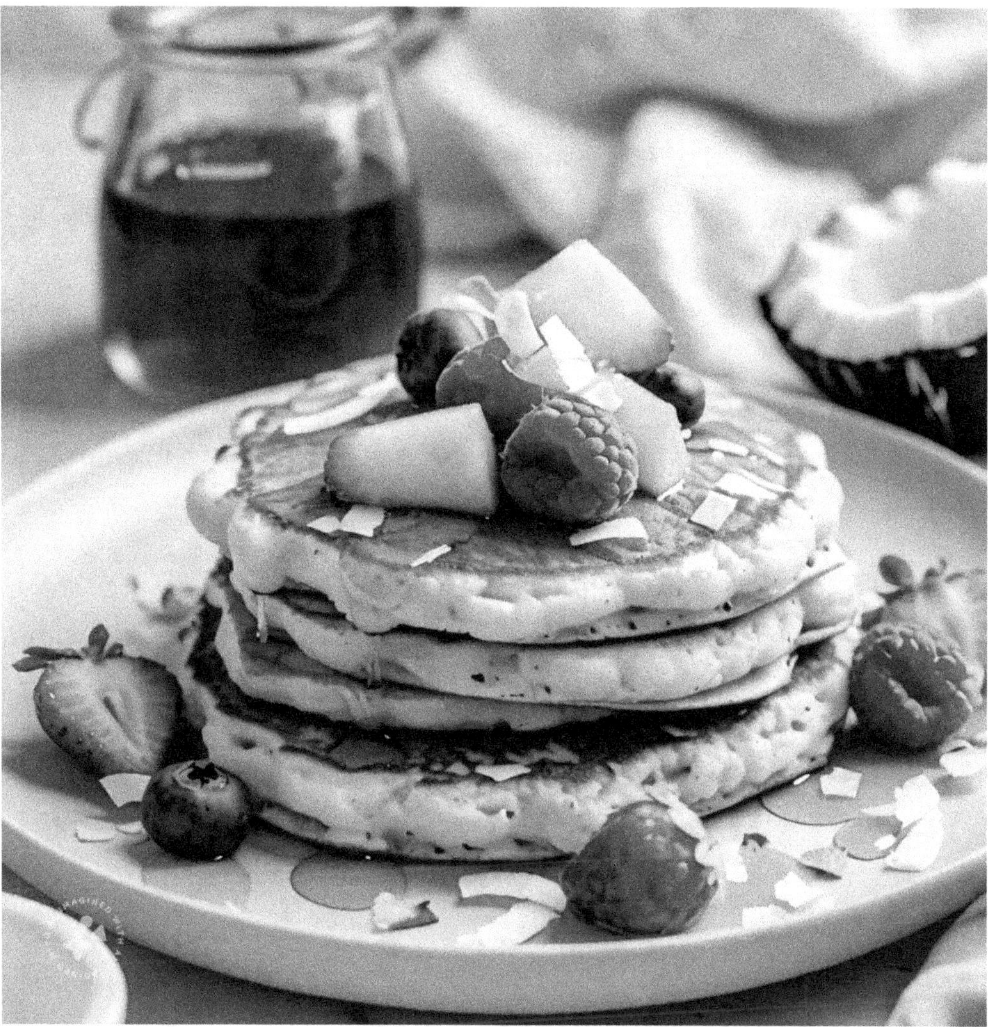

Ingredients:

- 1/4 cup coconut flour

- 4 large eggs

- 1/4 cup almond milk (unsweetened)

- 1 tablespoon coconut oil (melted)

- 1 teaspoon vanilla extract

- 1/2 teaspoon baking powder

- 1/4 teaspoon salt

- 1 tablespoon sweetener of choice (optional, like stevia or erythritol)

- Fresh berries (for topping)

- Butter or oil (for cooking)

Instructions:

1. **Prepare the Batter:**

  - In a medium bowl, whisk the eggs until smooth.

  - Add the almond milk, melted coconut oil, and vanilla extract, and mix well.

  - In a separate bowl, sift together the coconut flour, baking powder, salt, and sweetener (if using).

  - Gradually add the dry ingredients to the wet mixture, whisking continuously to avoid lumps. Let the batter sit for a few minutes to thicken.

2. **Cook the Pancakes:**

  - Heat a non-stick pan or griddle over medium heat and lightly grease with butter or oil.

  - Pour about 2 tablespoons of batter per pancake onto the pan. Spread it out gently with the back of the spoon to form a small circle, as the batter is thicker than regular pancake batter.

  - Cook for about 2-3 minutes until bubbles form on the surface and the edges start to firm up.

  - Flip the pancakes carefully and cook for another 2-3 minutes until golden brown and cooked through.

3. **Serve:**

  - Stack the pancakes on a plate and top with fresh berries of your choice.

12. Keto Avocado Smoothie

This smoothie, which is high in healthy fats, helps people lose weight while also delivering a creamy, pleasant drink.

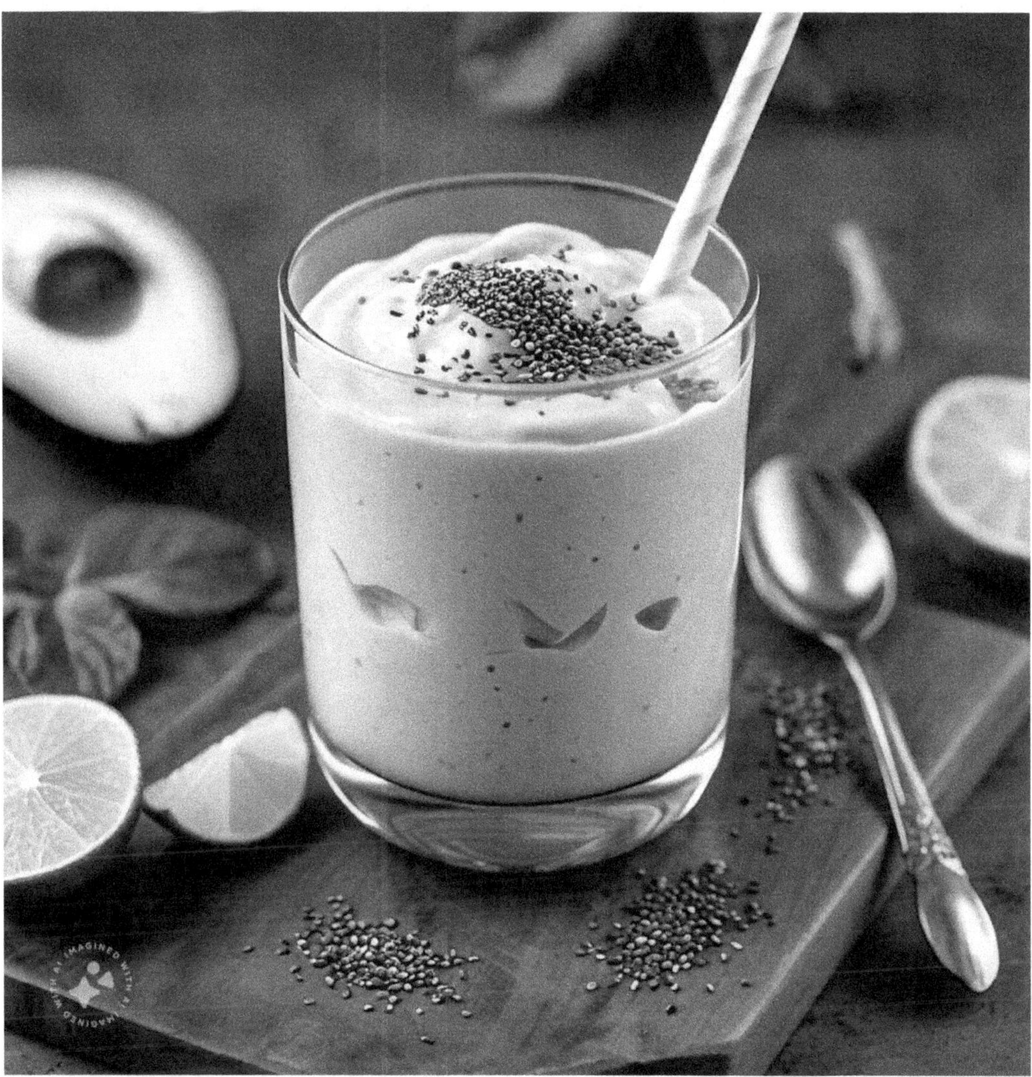

Ingredients:

- 1 ripe avocado, peeled and pitted

- 1 cup fresh spinach leaves

- 1 cup unsweetened coconut milk

- 1/2 cup water (or more for desired consistency)

- 1 tablespoon chia seeds (optional for extra fiber)

- 1/2 teaspoon vanilla extract (optional)

- 1-2 packets stevia (or sweetener of choice, adjust to taste)

- Ice cubes (optional, for a chilled smoothie)

Instructions:

1. **Prepare the Ingredients:**

   - Cut the avocado in half, remove the pit, and scoop the flesh into a blender.

   - Add the spinach, coconut milk, water, chia seeds (if using), vanilla extract, and stevia.

2. **Blend the Smoothie:**

   - Blend everything on high speed until smooth and creamy. If the smoothie is too thick, add more water or coconut milk, a little at a time, to reach your desired consistency.

3. **Add Ice (Optional):**

   - For a chilled smoothie, add a few ice cubes and blend again until well incorporated.

4. **Serve:**

   - Pour into a glass and enjoy immediately.

13. Keto BLT Salad

It's a tasty, low-carb salad with healthy fats and proteins from bacon and avocado that will keep you satisfied.

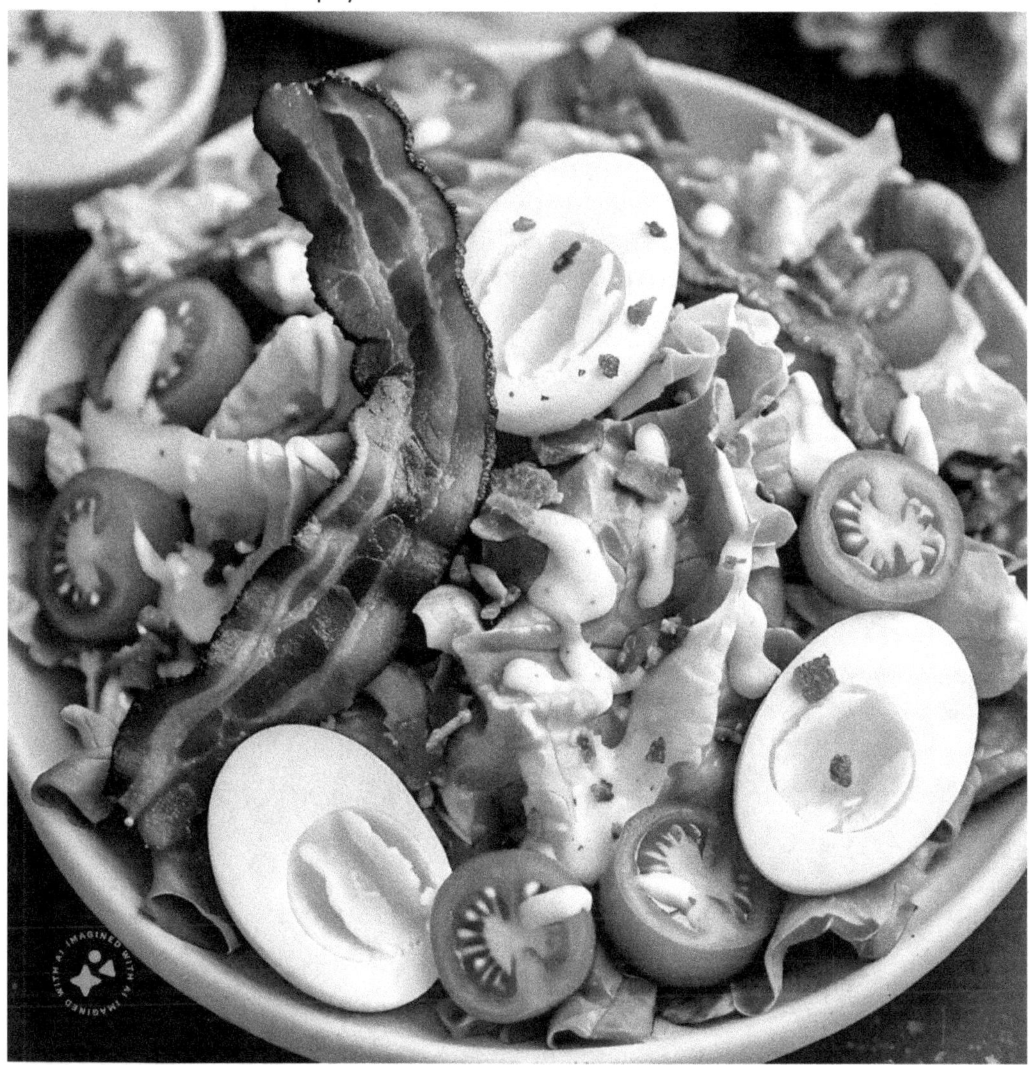

Ingredients:

- 4 cups romaine lettuce, chopped

- 6 slices bacon, cooked and crumbled

- 1 large tomato, diced

- 1 ripe avocado, diced

- 1/4 cup ranch dressing (store-bought or homemade)

- Salt and pepper, to taste

- Optional: 1 tablespoon chopped fresh chives or parsley for garnish

Instructions:

1. **Prepare the Bacon:**

   - Cook the bacon in a skillet over medium heat until crispy. Once done, transfer to a paper towel to drain, then crumble it into bite-sized pieces.

2.   **Assemble the Salad:**

   - In a large bowl, add the chopped romaine lettuce.

   - Top with the diced tomato, avocado, and crumbled bacon.

3. **Dress the Salad:**

   - Drizzle the ranch dressing over the salad and toss gently to combine all the ingredients.

4. **Season and Serve:**

   - Season with salt and pepper to taste.

   - Optionally, garnish with fresh chives or parsley for a burst of flavor.

14. Garlic Lemon Butter Scallops

Scallops are abundant in lean protein and low in calories, with garlic and lemon providing antioxidants and vitamins.

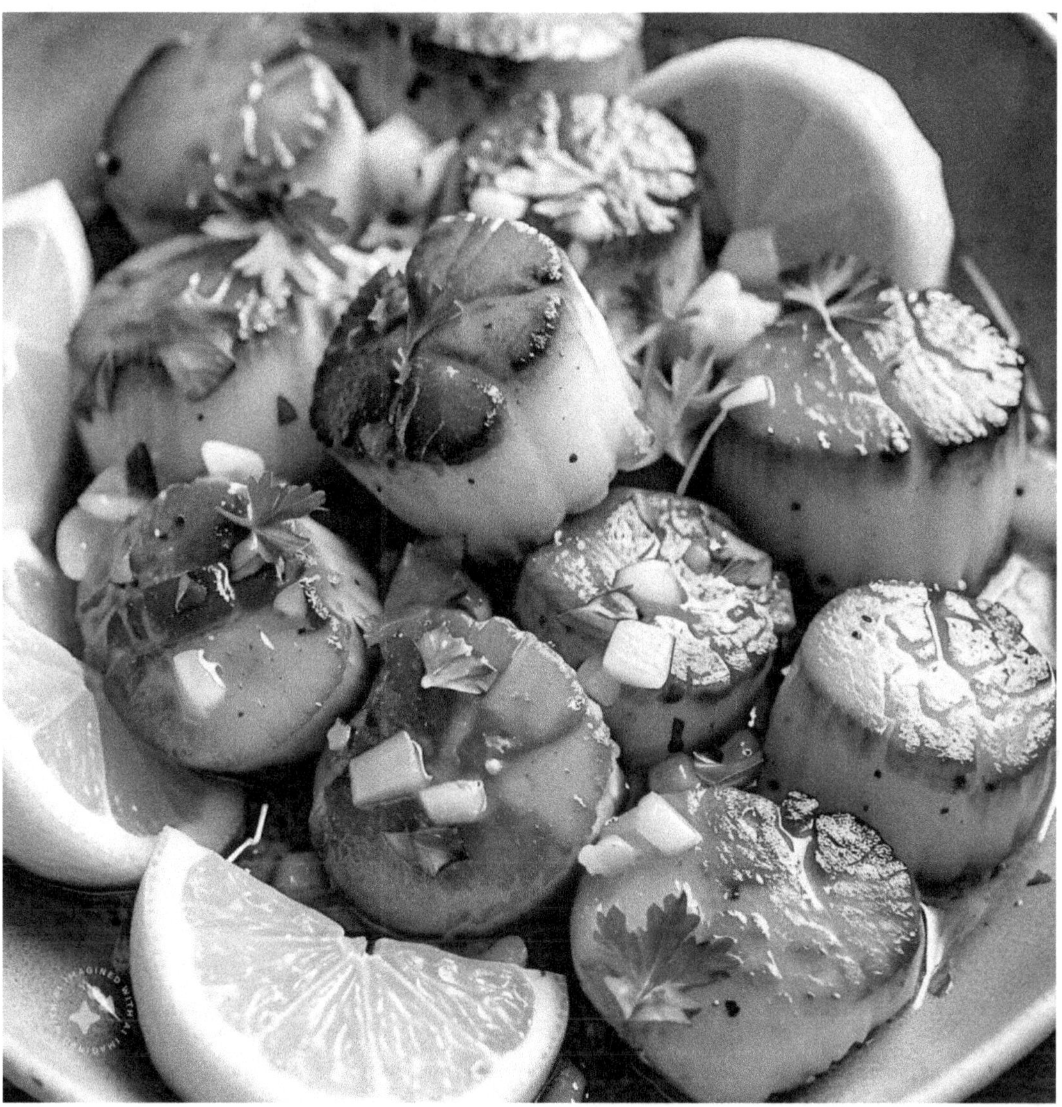

Ingredients:

- 450g (1 lb) sea scallops, patted dry

- 2 tablespoons unsalted butter

- 1 tablespoon olive oil

- 3 cloves garlic, minced

- 1/4 cup fresh lemon juice

- 1 tablespoon fresh parsley, chopped (optional, for garnish)

- Salt and pepper, to taste

- Lemon wedges (for serving)

Instructions:

1. **Prepare the Scallops:**

    - Pat the scallops dry with paper towels to remove excess moisture. Season both sides with salt and pepper.

2. **Sear the Scallops:**

    - Heat the olive oil in a large skillet over medium-high heat.

    - Once the pan is hot, add the scallops in a single layer, making sure not to overcrowd the pan. Sear the scallops for 2-3 minutes on each side until golden brown and opaque. Remove the scallops from the pan and set aside.

3. **Make the Garlic Lemon Butter Sauce:**

    - In the same pan, lower the heat to medium. Add the butter and let it melt.

    - Add the minced garlic and cook for 1 minute until fragrant.

    - Stir in the lemon juice, scraping up any browned bits from the pan. Let the sauce simmer for 1-2 minutes to thicken slightly.

4. **Return Scallops to the Pan:**

    - Return the seared scallops to the pan and spoon the garlic lemon butter sauce over them. Cook for an additional minute to heat through.

5. **Serve:**

    - Transfer the scallops to a serving plate, drizzle with the remaining sauce, and garnish with chopped parsley and lemon wedges.

15. Cauliflower Fried Rice

Cauliflower, a low-carb alternative to regular rice, has vitamins C and K, which aid digestion and weight loss.

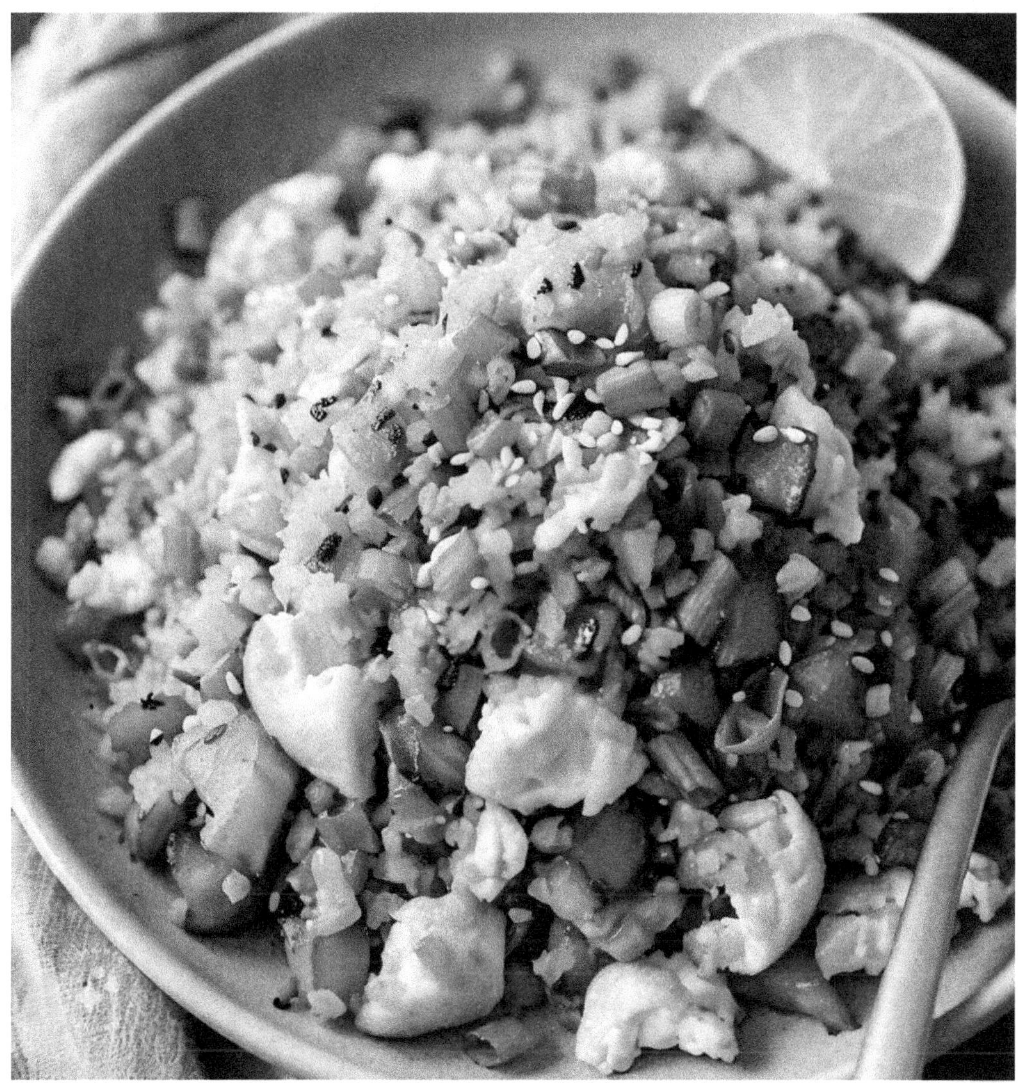

Ingredients:

- 4 cups riced cauliflower (store-bought or homemade)

- 2 large eggs, lightly beaten

- 1/2 cup peas (fresh or frozen)

- 1/2 cup carrots, diced

- 2 green onions, chopped

- 2 cloves garlic, minced

- 3 tablespoons soy sauce (or tamari for gluten-free)

- 1 tablespoon sesame oil

- 1 tablespoon olive oil

- Salt and pepper, to taste

- Optional: 1 teaspoon grated ginger or red pepper flakes for extra flavor

Instructions:

1. **Prepare the Vegetables:**

   - If using frozen peas, thaw them ahead of time. Dice the carrots and chop the green onions.

2. **Scramble the Eggs:**

   - Heat 1 tablespoon of olive oil in a large pan or wok over medium heat.

   - Add the beaten eggs, scrambling them until fully cooked. Once done, remove from the pan and set aside.

3. **Stir-fry the Vegetables:**

   - In the same pan, add the sesame oil and sauté the garlic for 1 minute until fragrant.

   - Add the diced carrots and cook for 3-4 minutes until slightly tender.

   - Stir in the peas and green onions, cooking for another 2 minutes.

4. **Add the Cauliflower Rice:**

   - Add the riced cauliflower to the pan, stirring everything together.

   - Pour in the soy sauce and cook for 5-7 minutes, stirring occasionally, until the cauliflower is tender and lightly golden.

5. **Finish the Dish:**

   - Add the scrambled eggs back into the pan and stir to combine with the vegetables and cauliflower.

- Season with salt and pepper to taste, and garnish with additional green onions or red pepper flakes if desired.

6. Serve:

- Serve the **Cauliflower Fried Rice** hot as a low-carb, healthy alternative to traditional fried rice.

16. Keto Cloud Bread

A soft, carb-free bread alternative prepared with eggs and cream cheese, perfect for low-carb sandwiches.

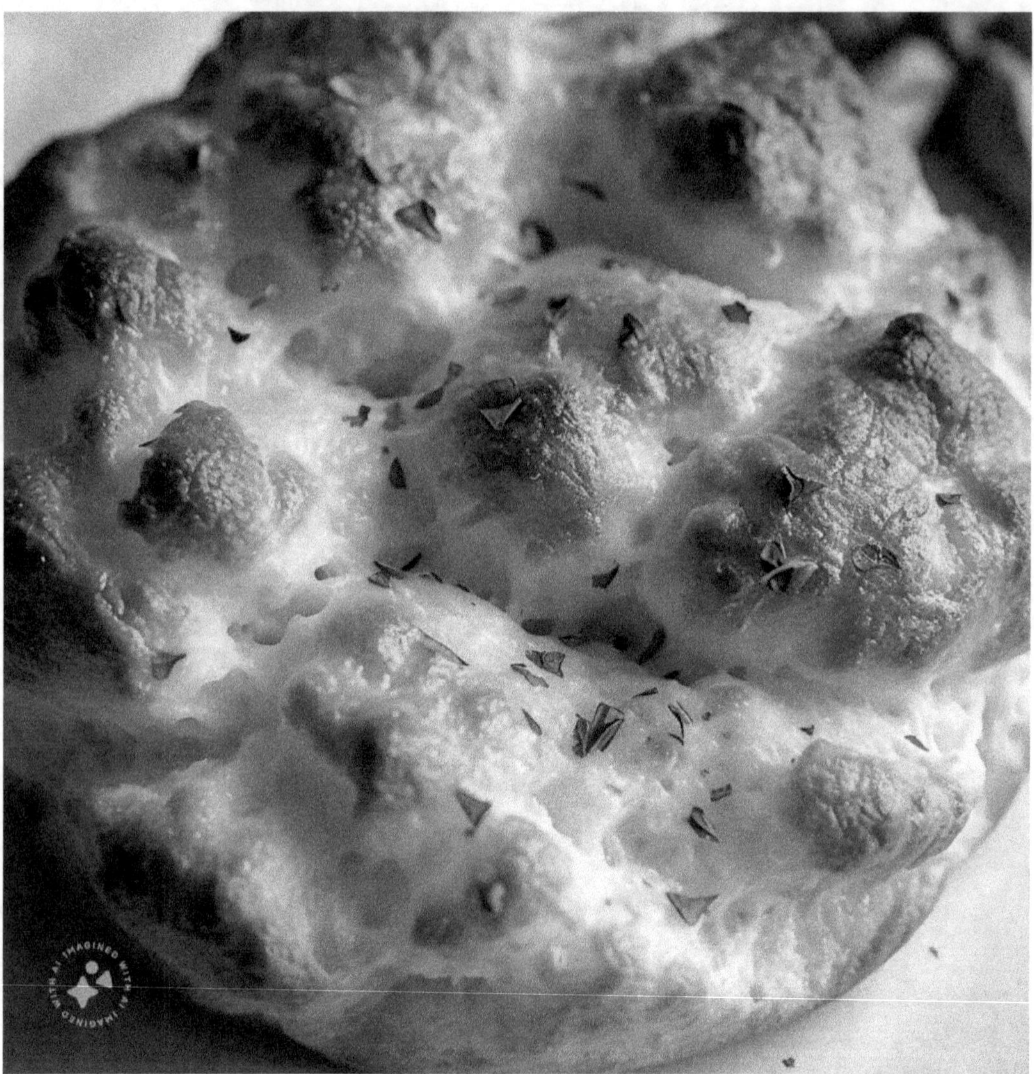

Ingredients:

- 3 large eggs, separated

- 3 tablespoons cream cheese, softened

- 1/4 teaspoon baking powder (or cream of tartar)

- 1/4 teaspoon salt (optional)

- 1/4 teaspoon garlic powder or herbs (optional, for added flavour)

Instructions:

1. Preheat the Oven:

   - Preheat your oven to 150°C (300°F) and line a baking sheet with parchment paper.

2. Prepare the Egg Mixture:

   - In a mixing bowl, whisk the egg whites with the baking powder (or cream of tartar) until stiff peaks form. This step is crucial to make the cloud bread light and fluffy.

   - In a separate bowl, beat the egg yolks and softened cream cheese until smooth and well combined. Add salt or garlic powder if desired.

3. Combine the Mixtures:

   - Gently fold the egg whites into the egg yolk mixture, being careful not to deflate the egg whites. Mix until just combined and fluffy.

4. Shape the Cloud Bread:

   - Using a spoon, scoop the batter onto the lined baking sheet, forming small, round shapes (about the size of a slice of bread).

   - Leave enough space between each round as they will spread slightly while baking.

5. Bake:

   - Bake in the preheated oven for 25-30 minutes, or until golden brown and firm to the touch.

6. Cool and Serve:

   - Let the cloud bread cool for a few minutes before removing from the baking sheet.

   - Serve immediately or store in an airtight container in the fridge.

17. Bacon-Wrapped Asparagus

Asparagus has fiber, vitamins A and K, and bacon provides protein and flavor, making it keto-friendly.

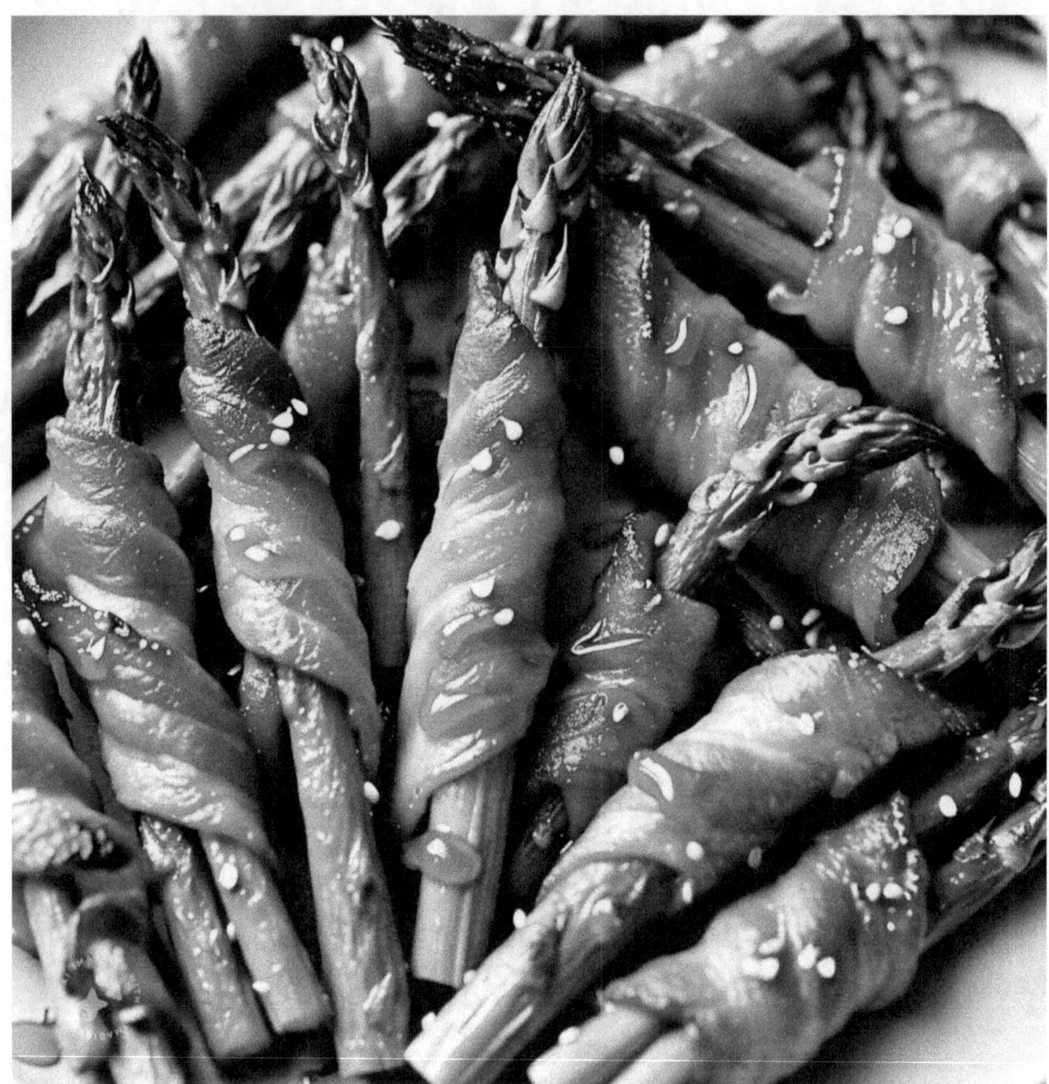

Ingredients:

- 450g (1 lb) fresh asparagus spears, trimmed

- 12 slices of bacon

- 2 tablespoons olive oil

- Salt and pepper, to taste

- Optional: 1 tablespoon grated Parmesan cheese (for garnish)

- Optional: Lemon wedges (for serving)

Instructions:

1. **Preheat the Oven:**

   - Preheat your oven to 200°C (400°F) and line a baking sheet with parchment paper or foil for easy clean up.

2. **Prepare the Asparagus:**

   - Trim the tough ends off the asparagus spears, ensuring they are about the same length for even cooking.

3. **Wrap the Asparagus:**

   - Take one slice of bacon and wrap it around each asparagus spear, starting from the bottom and spiraling up to the top. If the bacon is particularly long, you may want to cut it in half.

4. **Arrange on Baking Sheet:**

   - Place the bacon-wrapped asparagus on the prepared baking sheet in a single layer. Drizzle with olive oil and sprinkle with salt and pepper.

5. **Bake:**

   - Bake in the preheated oven for 20-25 minutes, or until the bacon is crispy and the asparagus is tender. You can broil for the last few minutes for extra crispiness.

6. Serve:

   - Remove from the oven and allow to cool slightly. Optionally, sprinkle with grated Parmesan cheese and serve with lemon wedges on the side.

18. Keto Chicken Tacos (Lettuce Wraps)

Lettuce wraps include fewer carbohydrates, yet the filling is high in protein, keeping you active and in ketosis.

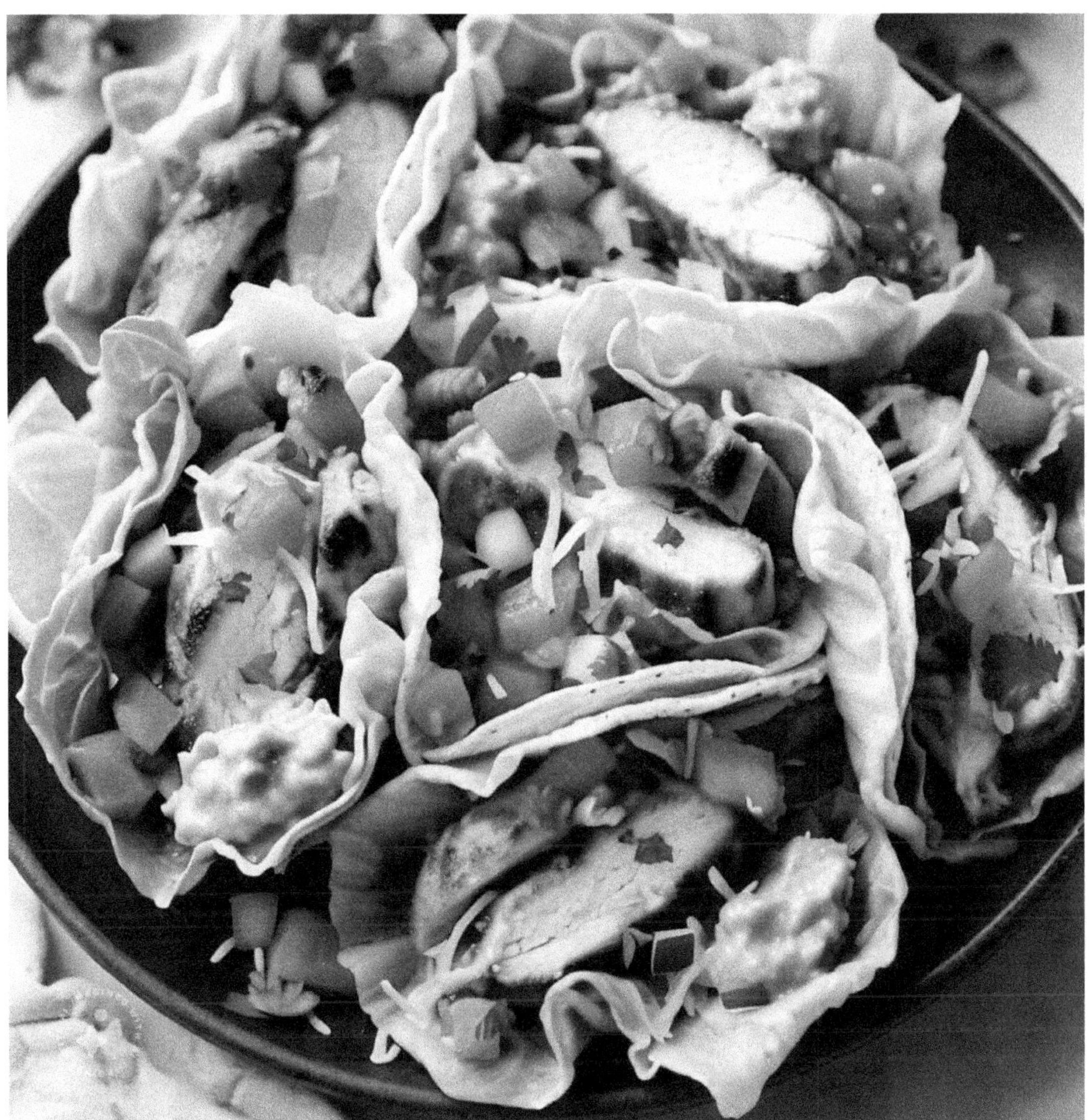

Ingredients:

- 450g (1 lb) chicken breast, grilled and sliced

- 1 tablespoon olive oil

- 1 teaspoon taco seasoning (or to taste)

- 8 large lettuce leaves (Romaine or Iceberg works well)

- 1 ripe avocado, mashed (for guacamole)

- 1/2 cup salsa (fresh or store-bought)

- 1/4 cup shredded cheese (optional)

- Fresh cilantro (optional, for garnish)

- Lime wedges (for serving)

- Salt and pepper, to taste

Instructions:

1. **Prepare the Chicken:**

   - Season the chicken breasts with olive oil, taco seasoning, salt, and pepper.

   - Grill the chicken over medium heat for 6-8 minutes on each side, or until fully cooked and juices run clear. Let it rest for a few minutes, then slice into strips.

2. **Prepare the Guacamole:**

   - In a bowl, mash the ripe avocado with a fork. Season with salt and lime juice to taste.

3. **Assemble the Tacos:**

   - Take a lettuce leaf and place a few slices of grilled chicken in the center.

   - Top with a generous dollop of guacamole and a spoonful of salsa. If desired, sprinkle with shredded cheese.

4. **Wrap and Serve:**

   - Fold the lettuce leaf over the filling like a taco and enjoy!

   - Garnish with fresh cilantro and serve with lime wedges on the side for extra zest.

19. Keto Cheeseburger Casserole

This dish is high in fats and protein, providing fullness while remaining low in carbs for keto diets.

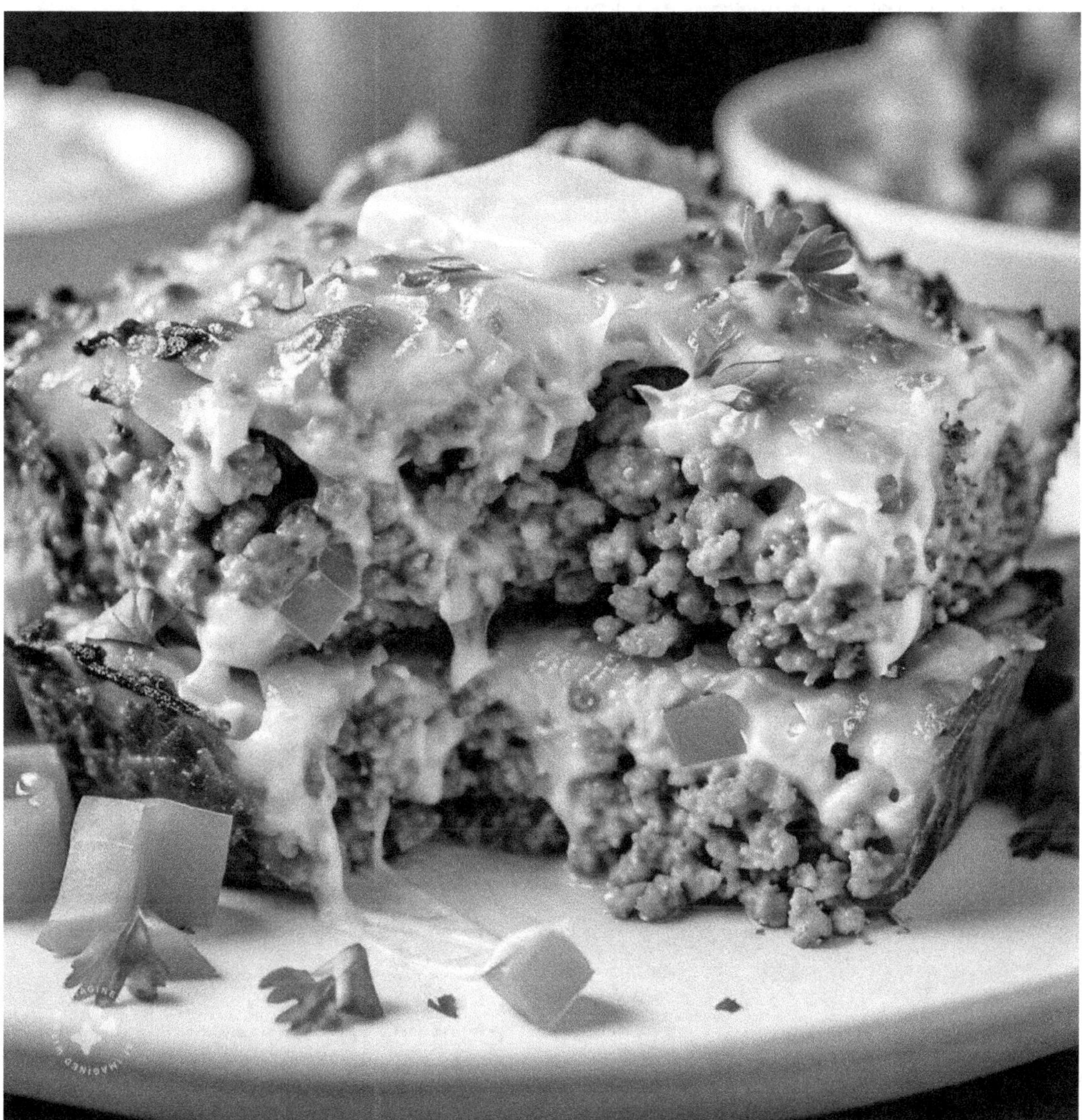

Ingredients:

- 450g (1 lb) ground beef

- 1 cup cream cheese, softened

- 1 cup shredded cheddar cheese

- 1/2 cup pickles, chopped (dill or sweet, based on preference)

- 1/2 cup onion, diced

- 2 cloves garlic, minced

- 1 tablespoon Worcestershire sauce

- 1 teaspoon mustard (yellow or Dijon)

- Salt and pepper, to taste

- 1 teaspoon paprika (optional, for extra flavour)

- Fresh parsley, chopped (for garnish)

Instructions:

1. **Preheat the Oven:**

   - Preheat your oven to 180°C (350°F) and grease a 9x9-inch (or similar size) baking dish.

2. **Cook the Ground Beef:**

   - In a large skillet, cook the ground beef over medium heat until browned. Drain any excess fat.

   - Add the diced onion and minced garlic, cooking until the onion is soft and translucent, about 3-4 minutes.

3. **Combine Ingredients:**

   - Reduce the heat to low and stir in the softened cream cheese until melted and well combined.

   - Add Worcestershire sauce, mustard, chopped pickles, salt, pepper, and paprika (if using). Mix until everything is evenly distributed.

4. **Transfer to Baking Dish:**

   - Pour the beef mixture into the prepared baking dish. Spread it out evenly.

   - Top with shredded cheddar cheese.

5. **Bake:**

   - Bake in the preheated oven for 20-25 minutes, or until the cheese is bubbly and golden.

6. **Serve:**

   - Remove from the oven and let it cool for a few minutes before serving.

   - Garnish with chopped fresh parsley if desired.

20. Broccoli and Cheddar Soup

Broccoli provides fiber and minerals, while cheddar adds important fats to this satisfying keto-friendly soup.

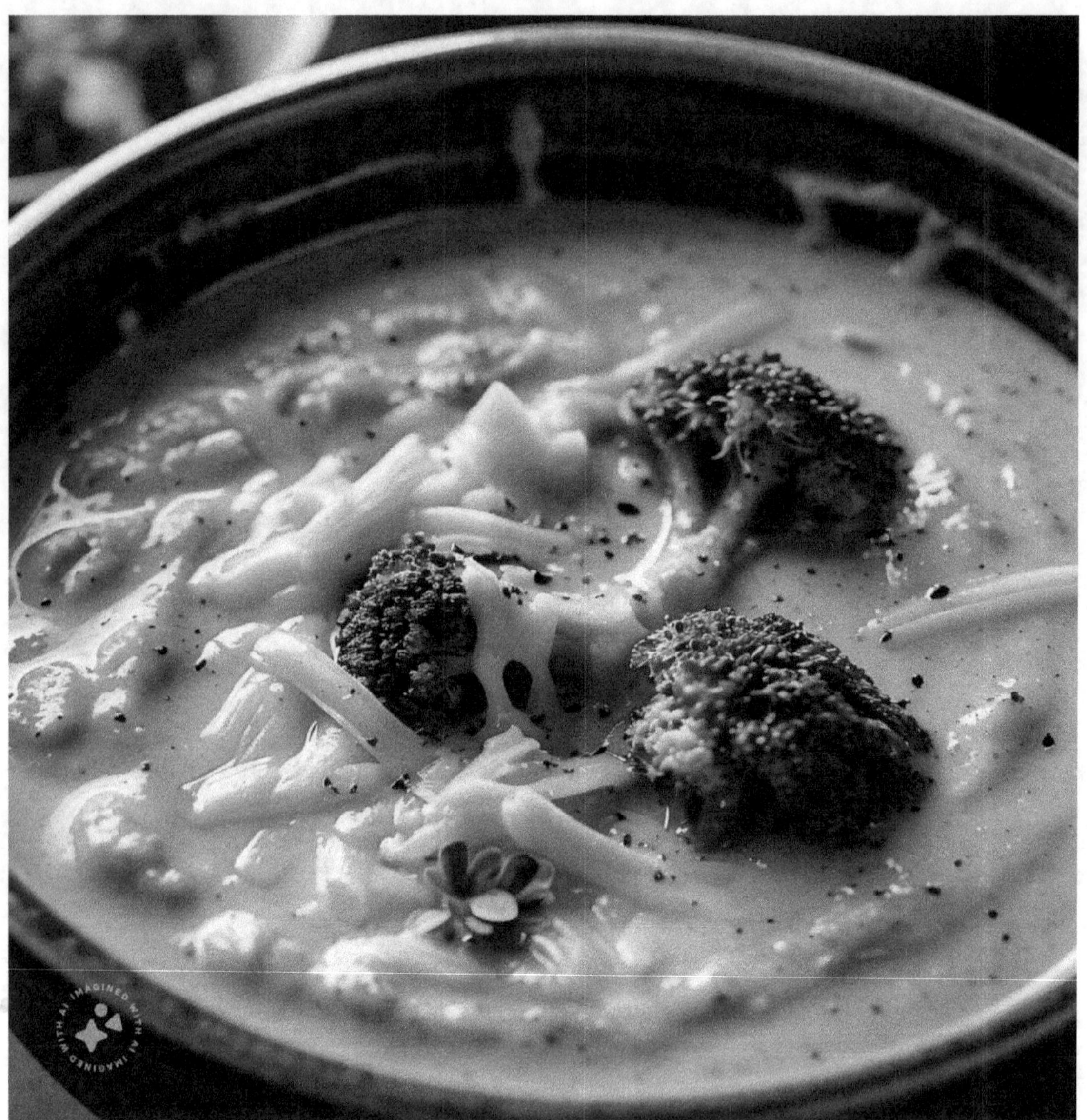

Ingredients:

- 4 cups broccoli florets

- 2 cups chicken or vegetable broth

- 1 cup heavy cream

- 1 1/2 cups shredded cheddar cheese

- 1/2 cup onion, diced

- 2 cloves garlic, minced

- 2 tablespoons butter

- Salt and pepper, to taste

- 1/4 teaspoon ground nutmeg (optional, for added flavour)

- Extra shredded cheddar cheese (for garnish)

- Fresh parsley or chives (for garnish)

Instructions:

1. **Prepare the Broccoli:**

   - Steam or blanch the broccoli florets for 3-4 minutes until tender. Set aside.

2. **Sauté Onion and Garlic:**

   - In a large pot, melt the butter over medium heat. Add the diced onion and sauté until soft and translucent, about 4-5 minutes.

   - Add the minced garlic and cook for another 1 minute until fragrant.

3. **Cook the Soup Base:**

   - Pour in the chicken or vegetable broth and bring to a simmer.

   - Add the cooked broccoli to the pot and simmer for 5-7 minutes, allowing the flavors to blend.

4. **Blend the Soup:**

- Using an immersion blender, blend the soup until smooth and creamy. If you don't have an immersion blender, transfer the soup in batches to a regular blender and blend until smooth.

5. **Add Cream and Cheese:**

- Stir in the heavy cream and bring the soup back to a simmer.

- Gradually add the shredded cheddar cheese, stirring constantly until the cheese is melted and the soup is creamy.

6. **Season and Serve:**

- Season with salt, pepper, and nutmeg (if using) to taste.

- Serve hot, garnished with extra shredded cheddar and fresh parsley or chives.

21. Quinoa Salad with Chickpeas and Feta

Quinoa Salad with Chickpeas and Feta: This salad is high in protein and fiber, which promotes digestive health and keeps you satisfied for longer.

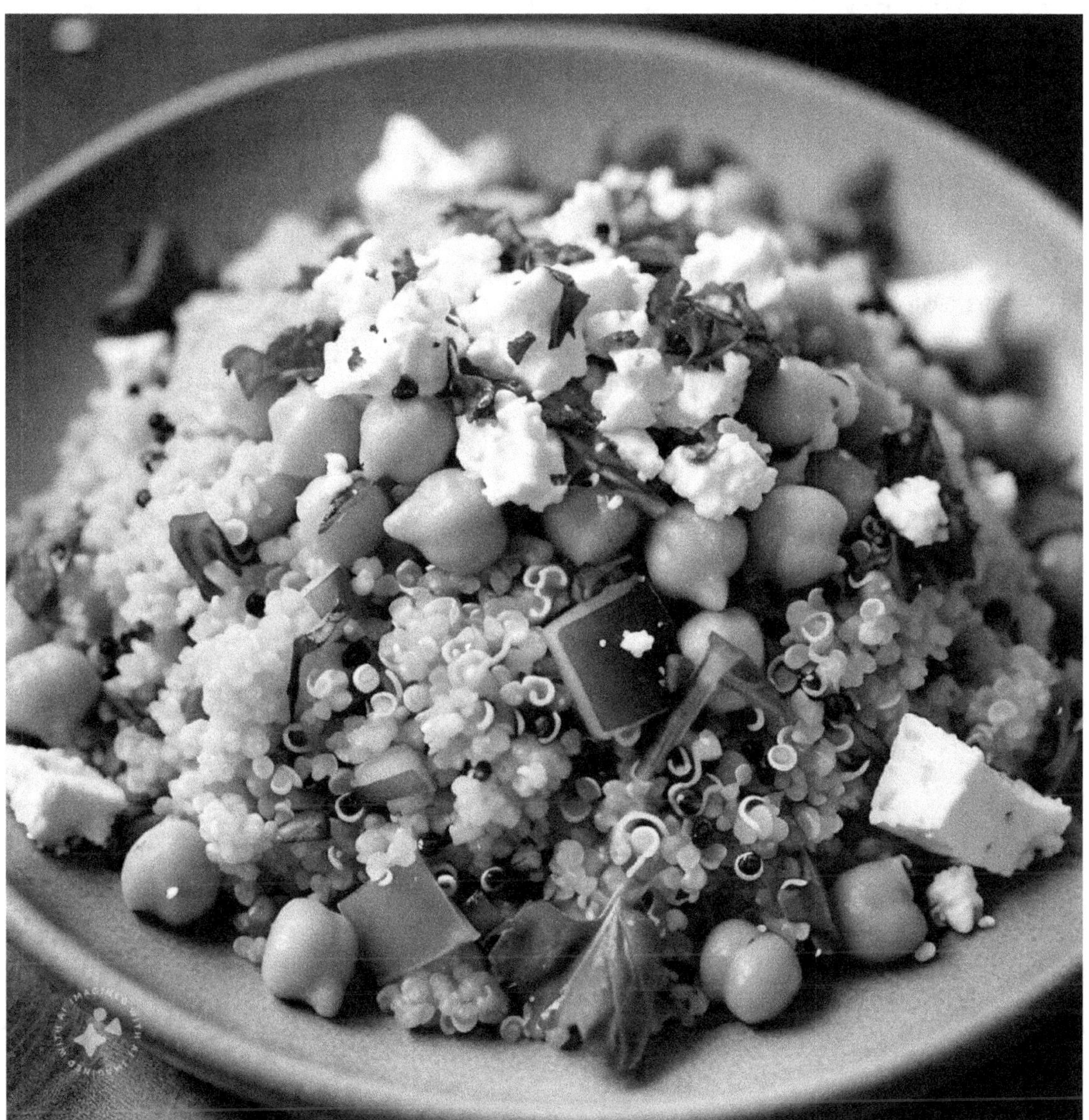

Ingredients:

- 1 cup quinoa

- 1 can (15 oz) chickpeas, drained and rinsed

- 1 cucumber, diced

- 1/2 cup crumbled feta cheese

- 2 tbsp olive oil

- 1 tbsp lemon juice

- Salt and pepper to taste

- Fresh parsley for garnish (optional)

Instructions:

1. Cook the quinoa:

Rinse the quinoa under cold water. In a medium saucepan, combine 1 cup of quinoa with 2 cups of water. Bring to a boil, then reduce the heat, cover, and simmer for 15 minutes, or until the quinoa is cooked. Fluff with a fork and let it cool.

2. Prepare the salad:

In a large bowl, combine the cooled quinoa, chickpeas, diced cucumber, and crumbled feta.

3. Make the dressing:

In a small bowl, whisk together the olive oil, lemon juice, salt, and pepper.

4. Toss the salad:

Pour the dressing over the quinoa mixture and toss until everything is well combined.

5. Serve:

Garnish with fresh parsley if desired, and serve chilled or at room temperature.

22. Sweet Potato and black bean Taco:

Sweet potatoes are high in fiber and vitamins, but chicken contains lean protein that promotes muscular growth.

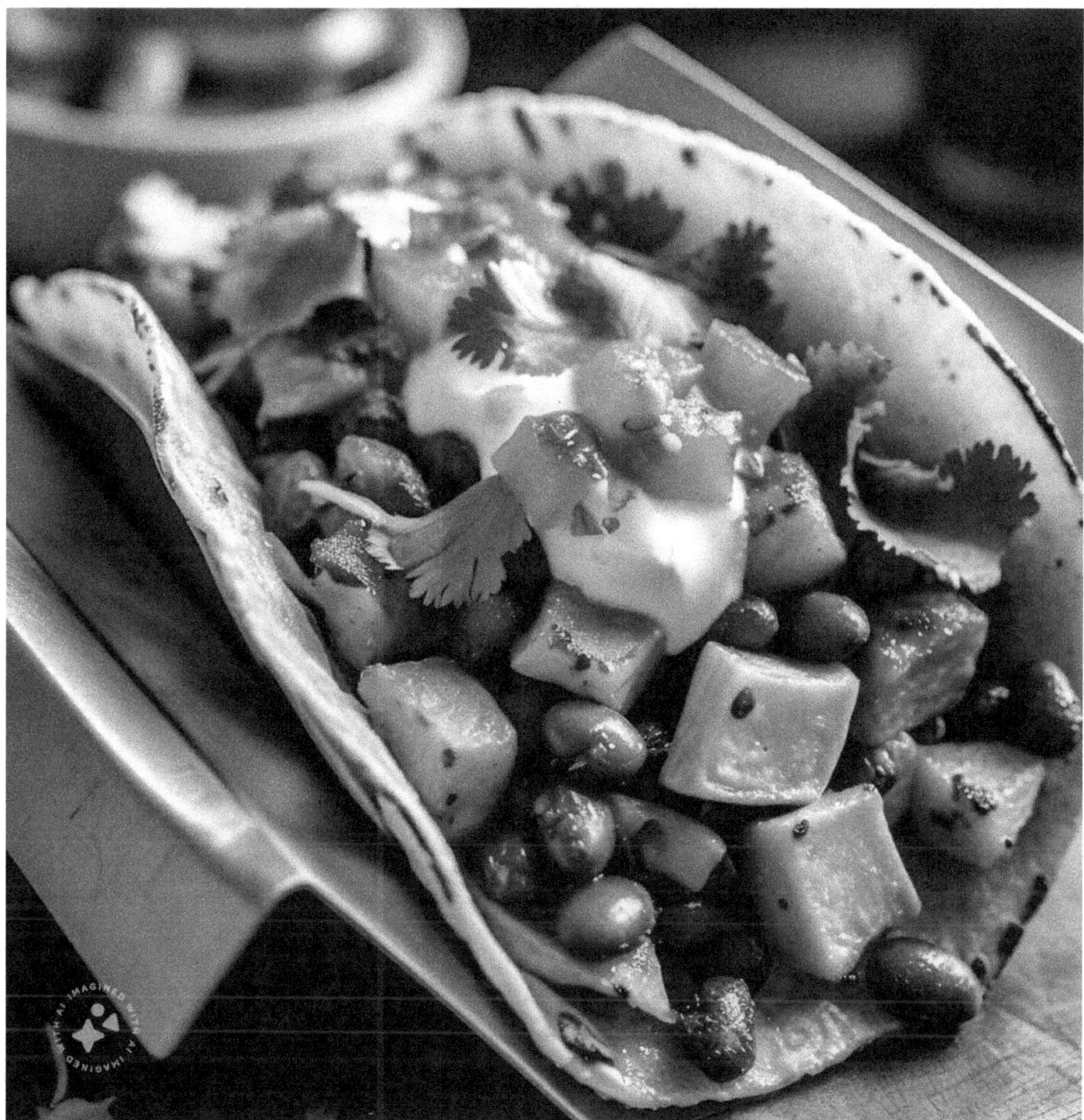

Ingredients:

- 2 medium sweet potatoes, peeled and diced

- 1 can (15 oz) black beans, drained and rinsed

- 1 tablespoon olive oil

- 1 teaspoon cumin

- 1 teaspoon smoked paprika

- 1/2 teaspoon chili powder

- Salt and pepper, to taste

- 8 small corn tortillas

- 1/2 cup red onion, diced

- 1/4 cup fresh cilantro, chopped

- 1 avocado, sliced

- 1 lime, cut into wedges

- Salsa, for serving (optional)

Instructions:

Preheat the oven:

 Set it to 400°F (200°C).

Roast the sweet potatoes:

Toss diced sweet potatoes in olive oil, cumin, paprika, chili powder, salt, and pepper. Spread them on a baking sheet and roast for 20-25 minutes until tender and slightly crispy.

1. **Heat the beans:**

While the sweet potatoes are roasting, warm the black beans in a small saucepan over low heat, adding salt and pepper to taste.

2. **Prepare the tortillas:**

Warm the corn tortillas in a dry skillet over medium heat for 1-2 minutes on each side.

3. **Assemble the tacos:**

Divide the roasted sweet potatoes and black beans among the tortillas. Top with diced red onion, cilantro, and avocado slices.

23. Spaghetti Bolognese

This classic comfort dish contains protein from ground beef and fiber from the sauce, but use low-carb pasta.

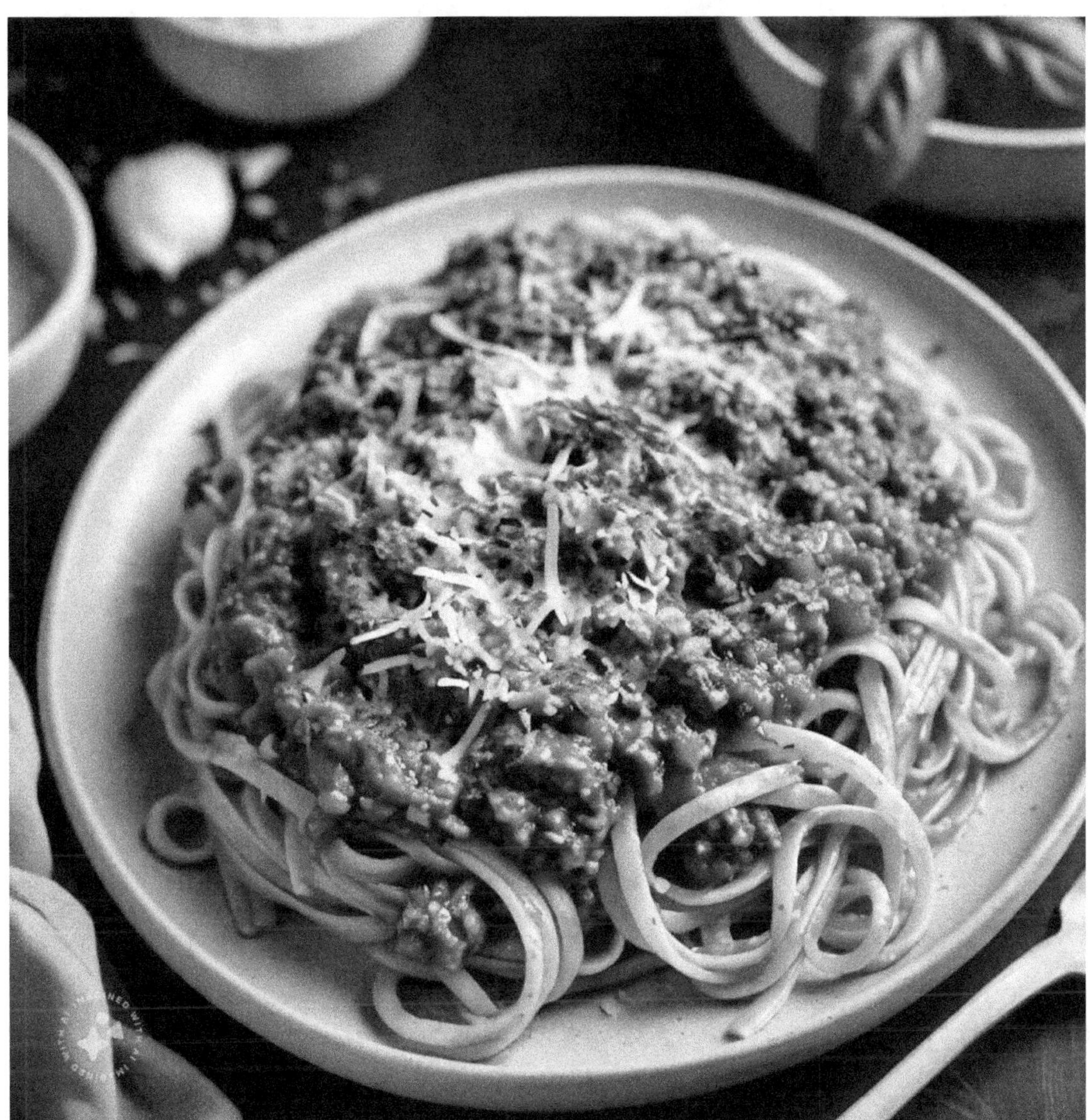

Ingredients:

- 400g whole wheat spaghetti

- 500g ground beef or turkey

- 1 onion, finely chopped

- 2 cloves garlic, minced

- 1 carrot, grated

- 1 celery stalk, finely chopped

- 1 can (400g) diced tomatoes

- 2 tablespoons tomato paste

- 1/2 cup beef or vegetable broth

- 1 teaspoon dried oregano

- 1 teaspoon dried basil

- 1/2 teaspoon chili flakes (optional)

- Salt and pepper, to taste

- 2 tablespoons olive oil

- Fresh parsley or basil, for garnish

- Grated Parmesan cheese, for serving

Instructions:

1. **Cook the pasta:**

Bring a large pot of salted water to a boil. Add the whole wheat spaghetti and cook according to package instructions. Drain and set aside.

2. **Sauté the vegetables:**

In a large skillet or pan, heat olive oil over medium heat. Add chopped onion, garlic, carrot, and celery, and sauté for about 5-7 minutes until soft.

3. **Cook the meat:**

Add the ground beef or turkey to the pan. Cook until browned, breaking it up into small pieces with a spoon, about 8-10 minutes.

4. **Add tomatoes and seasonings:**

Stir in the diced tomatoes, tomato paste, broth, oregano, basil, chili flakes (if using), salt, and pepper. Bring the mixture to a simmer and cook for 15-20 minutes, stirring occasionally, until the sauce thickens.

5. **Combine with pasta:**

Toss the cooked spaghetti with the Bolognese sauce until evenly coated.

6. **Serve:**

Garnish with fresh parsley or basil and grated Parmesan cheese.

24. Pasta Primavera

A vibrant dish with veggies that contains important vitamins, fiber, and antioxidants, served with whole grain pasta.

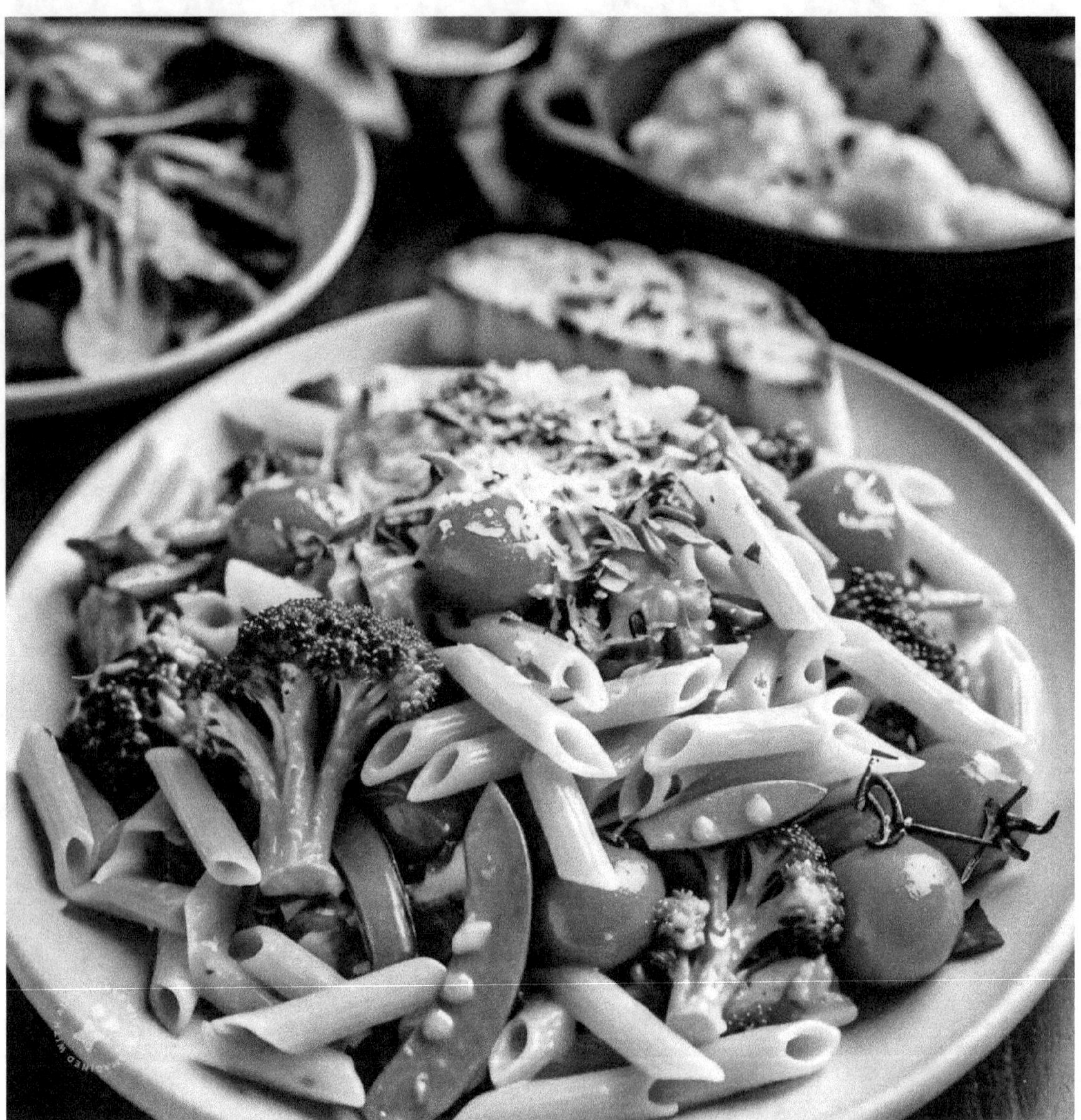

Ingredients:

- 400g whole grain pasta (penne or fusilli)

- 1 zucchini, sliced

- 1 bell pepper, sliced

- 1 carrot, julienned

- 1 cup cherry tomatoes, halved

- 1/2 cup broccoli florets

- 2 cloves garlic, minced

- 3 tablespoons olive oil

- 1 teaspoon dried oregano

- 1/2 teaspoon red pepper flakes (optional)

- Salt and pepper, to taste

- Fresh basil or parsley, chopped (for garnish)

- Grated Parmesan cheese, for serving

Instructions:

1. **Cook the pasta:**

Bring a large pot of salted water to a boil. Add the whole grain pasta and cook according to the package instructions. Drain and set aside.

2. **Sauté the vegetables:**

In a large skillet, heat olive oil over medium heat. Add garlic and sauté for about 30 seconds until fragrant. Add the zucchini, bell pepper, carrot, broccoli, and cherry tomatoes. Sauté for 5-7 minutes, stirring occasionally, until the vegetables are tender but still crisp.

3. **Season the vegetables:**

Stir in the dried oregano, red pepper flakes (if using), salt, and pepper. Cook for an additional 2 minutes to let the flavors blend.

4. **Combine with pasta:**

Toss the cooked pasta with the sautéed vegetables until everything is well combined.

5. **Serve:**

Garnish with fresh basil or parsley and sprinkle with grated Parmesan cheese.

25. Chicken Pita Wraps

Chicken provides lean protein, and whole wheat pita adds fiber, resulting in a balanced and enjoyable lunch.

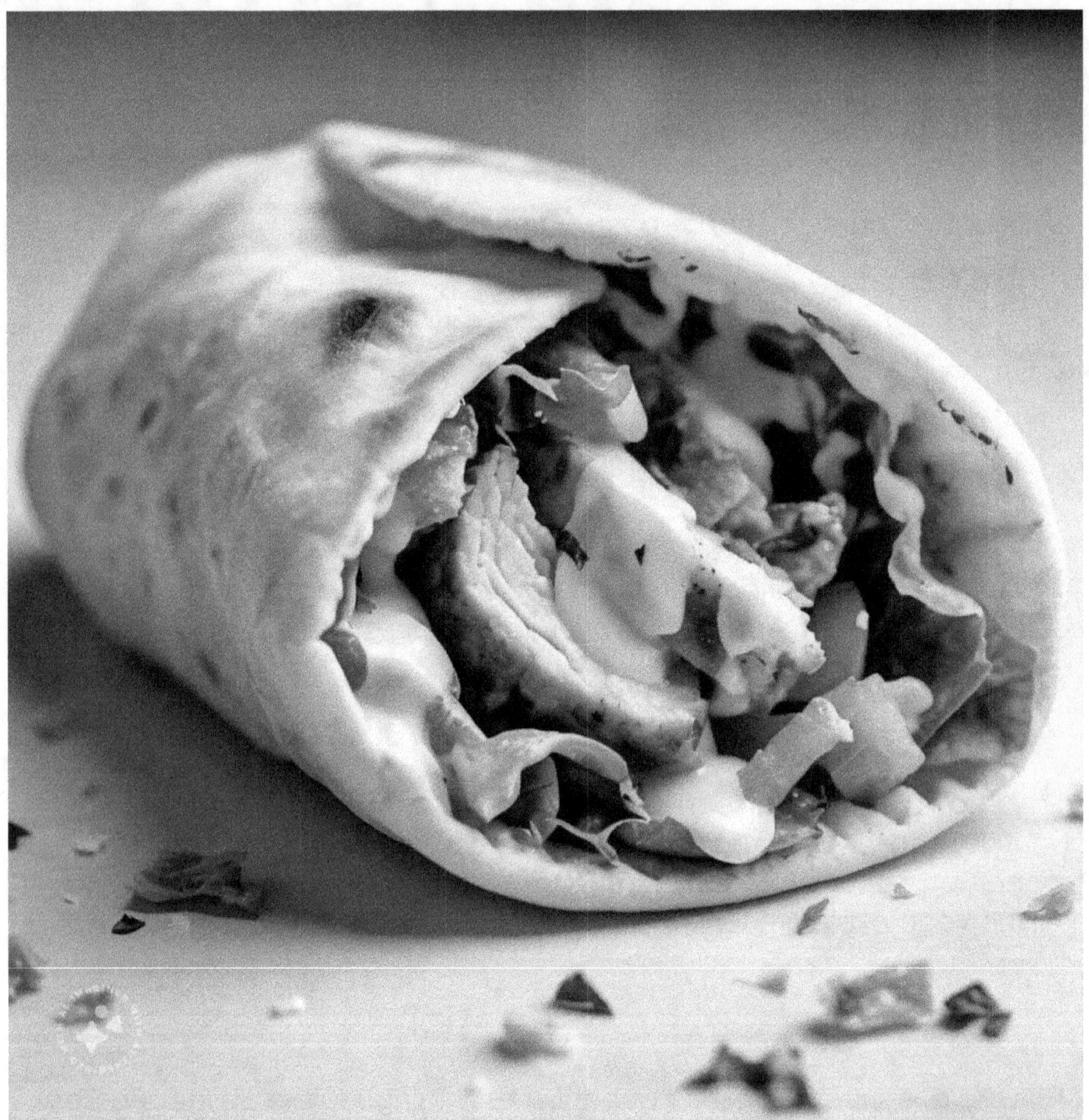

Ingredients:

- 2 whole wheat pita breads

- 2 chicken breasts, boneless and skinless

- 2 tablespoons olive oil

- 1 teaspoon paprika

- 1 teaspoon cumin

- 1/2 teaspoon garlic powder

- Salt and pepper, to taste

- 1/2 cup hummus

- 1/2 cucumber, thinly sliced

- 1 cup fresh spinach leaves

- 1/4 cup red onion, thinly sliced

- 1 tablespoon lemon juice

- Fresh parsley, chopped (optional)

Instructions:

1. **Marinate the chicken:**

In a bowl, mix olive oil, paprika, cumin, garlic powder, salt, and pepper. Coat the chicken breasts with the marinade and let them sit for 15-20 minutes.

2. **Grill the chicken:**

Preheat a grill or grill pan over medium heat. Grill the marinated chicken for 6-8 minutes per side, or until fully cooked and no longer pink in the center. Once cooked, let the chicken rest for a few minutes, then slice it into strips.

3. **Prepare the pita:**

Warm the whole wheat pita breads in a dry skillet or oven for 1-2 minutes.

4. **Assemble the wraps:**

Spread a generous amount of hummus inside each pita. Add sliced chicken, cucumber, spinach, and red onion. Drizzle with a bit of lemon juice for extra flavor.

5. **Serve:**

Garnish with fresh parsley, if desired, and serve the chicken pita wraps warm.

26. Oven-Roasted Potatoes and Brussels Sprouts

This recipe is high in fiber and vitamins, which promote digestive health and reduce inflammation.

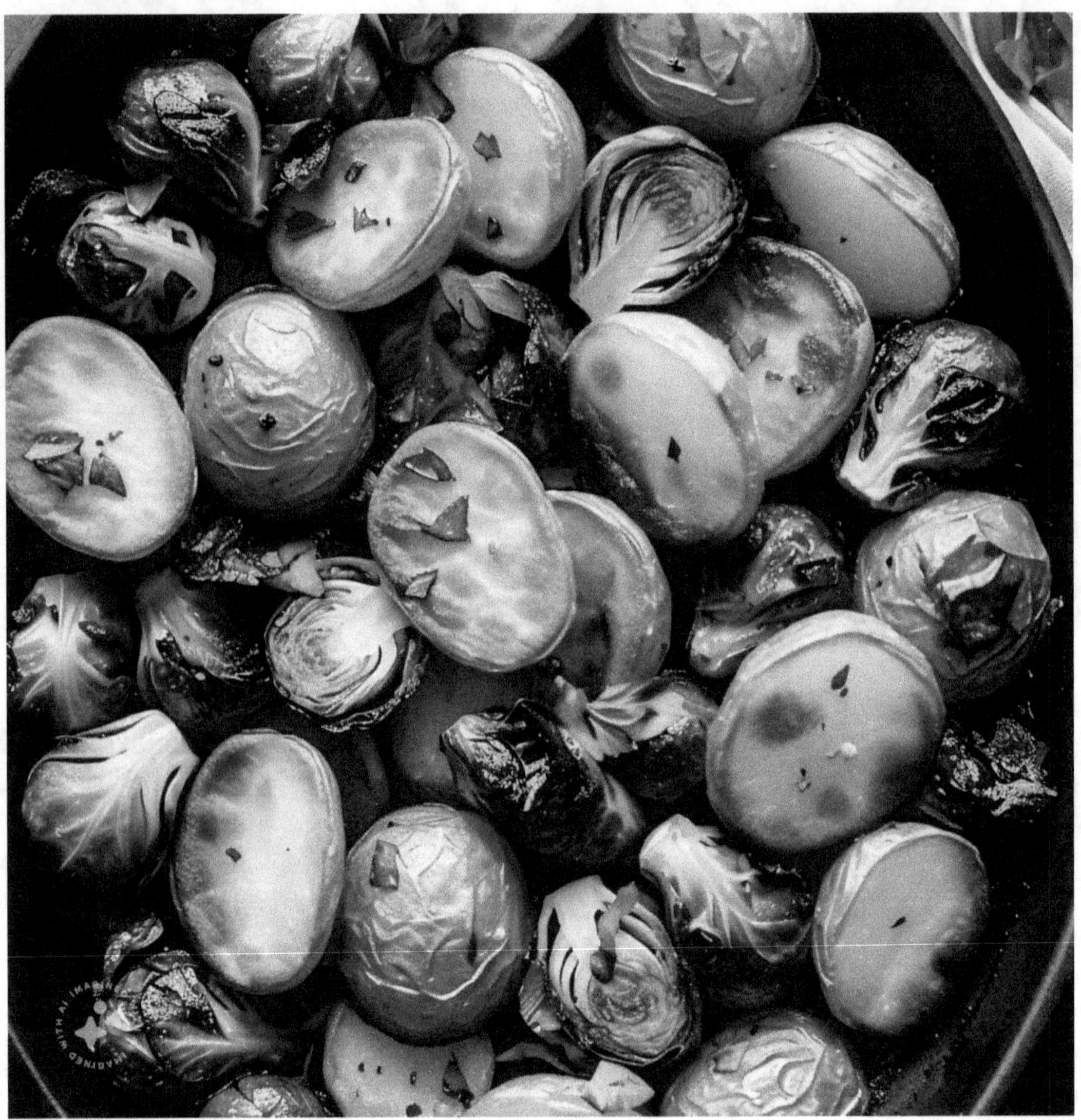

Ingredients:

- 500g baby potatoes, halved

- 400g Brussels sprouts, trimmed and halved

- 3 tablespoons olive oil

- 3 cloves garlic, minced

- 1 teaspoon dried rosemary (or 1 tablespoon fresh rosemary, chopped)

- 1/2 teaspoon paprika (optional)

- Salt and pepper, to taste

- Fresh parsley, chopped (for garnish)

Instructions:

1. **Preheat the oven:**

Set it to 200°C (400°F).

2. **Prepare the vegetables:**

In a large bowl, combine the halved potatoes and Brussels sprouts. Drizzle with olive oil, then add the minced garlic, rosemary, paprika (if using), salt, and pepper. Toss everything together until the vegetables are evenly coated.

3. **Roast the vegetables:**

Spread the potatoes and Brussels sprouts in a single layer on a baking sheet lined with parchment paper. Roast in the preheated oven for 25-30 minutes, stirring halfway through, until the potatoes are golden and crispy, and the Brussels sprouts are caramelized and tender.

4. **Serve:**

Remove from the oven and sprinkle with fresh parsley before serving.

27. Stuffed Bell Peppers

Bell peppers are abundant in vitamins C and A, and the filling contains protein, making this a well-balanced, low-carb lunch.

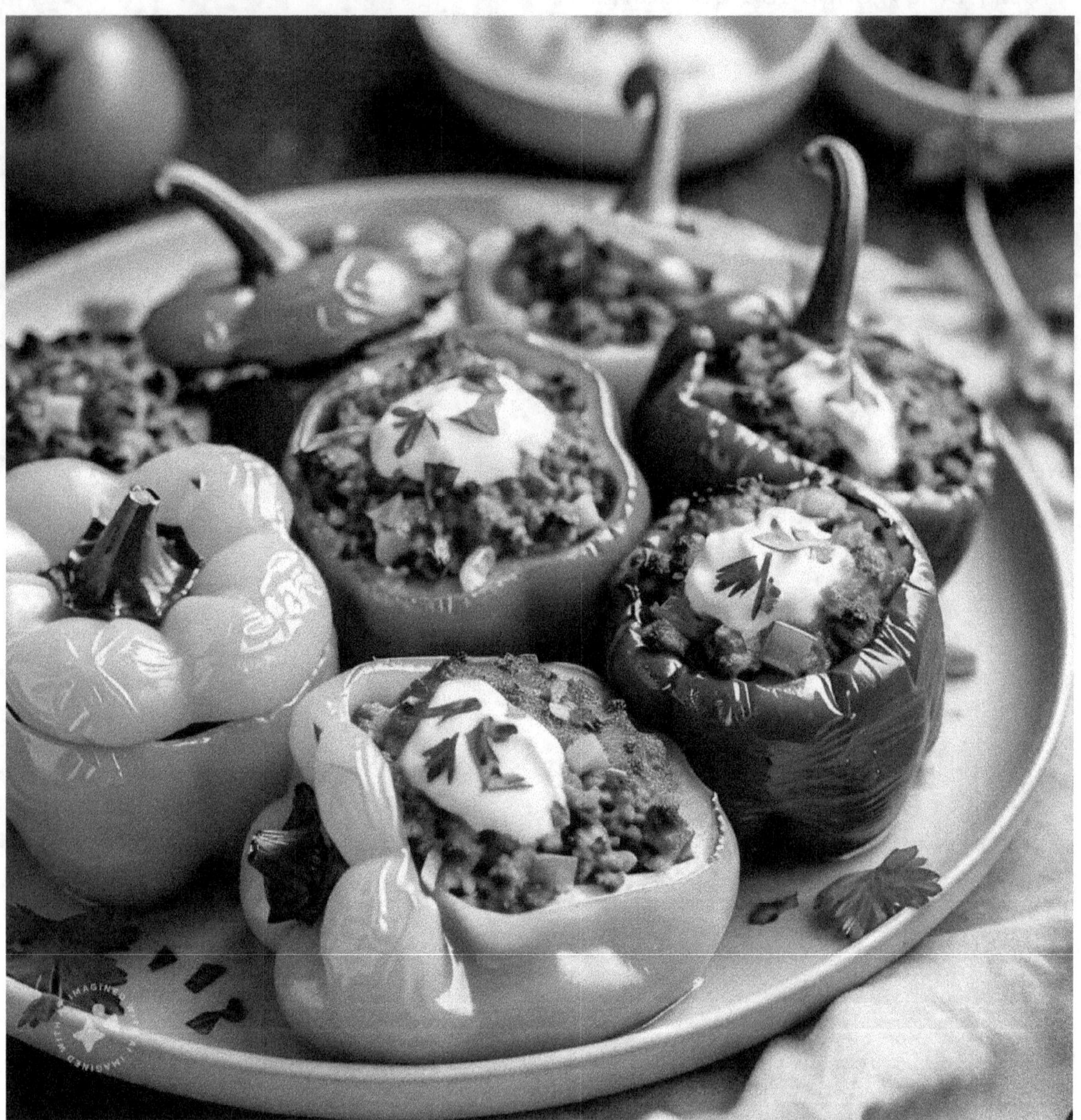

Ingredients:

- 4 large bell peppers (any color), tops cut off and seeds removed

- 250g ground beef

- 1 cup cooked rice

- 1 onion, finely chopped

- 2 cloves garlic, minced

- 1 can (400g) diced tomatoes

- 2 tablespoons tomato paste

- 1 teaspoon dried oregano

- 1 teaspoon paprika

- 1/2 teaspoon cumin

- Salt and pepper, to taste

- 1 tablespoon olive oil

- 1/2 cup shredded cheese (optional)

- Fresh parsley, chopped (for garnish)

Instructions:

1. **Preheat the oven:**

Set it to 180°C (350°F).

2. **Prepare the bell peppers:**

Cut off the tops of the bell peppers and remove the seeds and membranes. Set aside.

3. **Cook the filling:**

In a large skillet, heat olive oil over medium heat. Add the chopped onion and garlic, and sauté until softened, about 3-4 minutes. Add the ground beef, breaking it up with a spoon, and cook until browned. Drain any excess fat.

4. **Add the seasoning and rice:**

Stir in the diced tomatoes, tomato paste, oregano, paprika, cumin, salt, and pepper. Simmer for 5 minutes, then stir in the cooked rice.

5. **Stuff the peppers:**

Spoon the beef and rice mixture into each bell pepper, packing it in tightly. Place the stuffed peppers in a baking dish.

6. **Bake the peppers:**

Cover the dish with foil and bake in the preheated oven for 30 minutes. If using cheese, remove the foil after 30 minutes, sprinkle cheese on top of the peppers, and bake uncovered for an additional 10 minutes, or until the cheese is melted and bubbly.

7. **Serve:**

Garnish with fresh parsley and serve the stuffed bell peppers hot.

28. Vegetable Risotto

Made with fiber-rich veggies, this creamy meal provides a satisfying combination of carbohydrates and important nutrients.

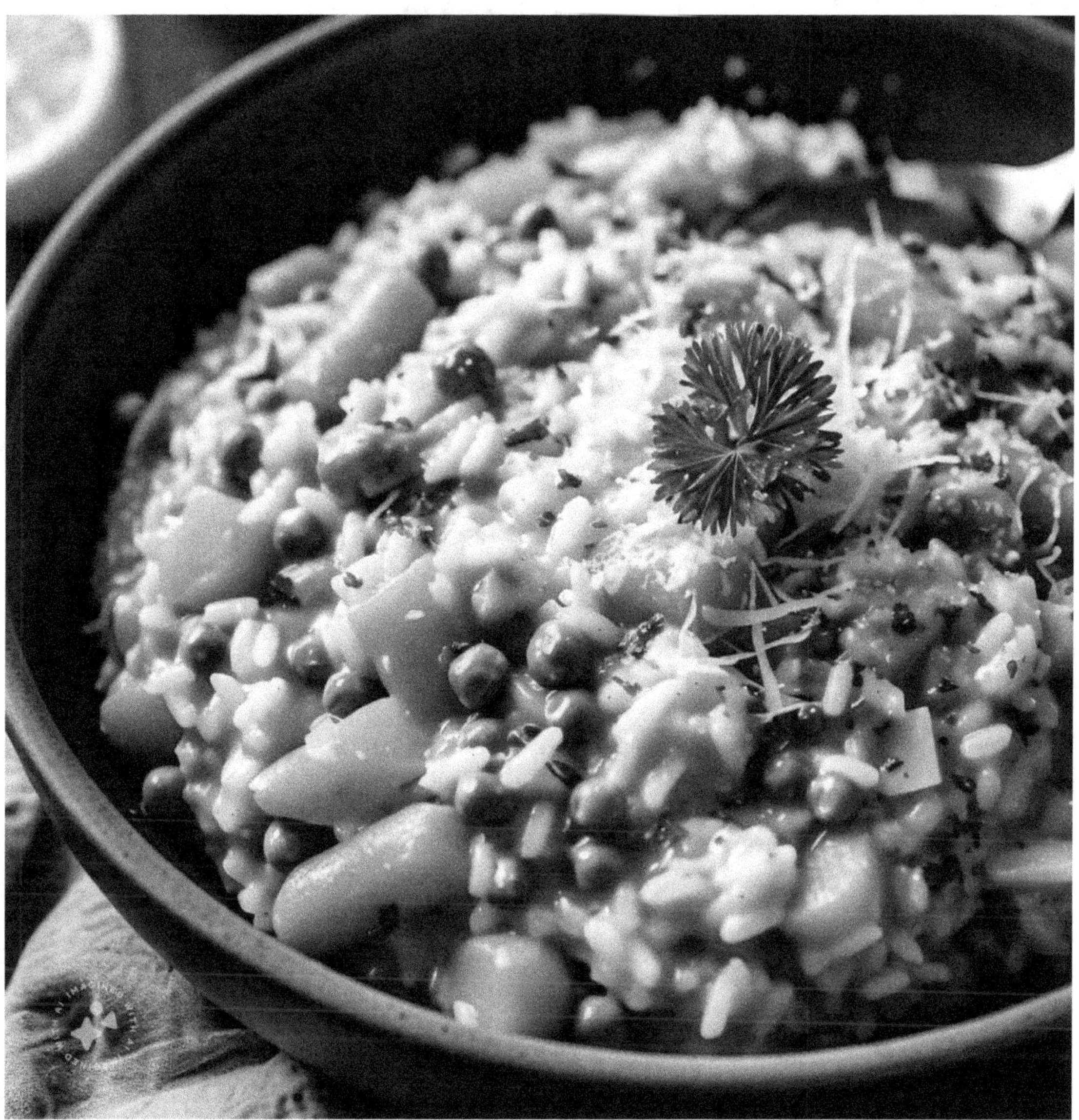

Ingredients:

- 1 ½ cups Arborio rice

- 1 tablespoon olive oil

- 1 onion, finely chopped

- 2 cloves garlic, minced

- 1/2 cup dry white wine (optional)

- 4 cups vegetable broth, warmed

- 1 cup peas (fresh or frozen)

- 1 cup asparagus, chopped

- 1/2 cup grated Parmesan cheese

- 2 tablespoons butter

- Salt and pepper, to taste

- Fresh parsley or basil, chopped (for garnish)

- Lemon zest (optional)

Instructions:

1. **Sauté the aromatics:**

In a large skillet or pot, heat olive oil over medium heat. Add the chopped onion and garlic, cooking for 3-4 minutes until soft and fragrant.

2. **Toast the rice:**

Stir in the Arborio rice, cooking for 1-2 minutes until it becomes slightly translucent around the edges.

3. **Add the wine:**

Pour in the white wine (if using) and cook until the liquid is absorbed, stirring constantly.

4. **Cook the risotto:**

Gradually add the warm vegetable broth, one ladle at a time, stirring continuously. Wait until the liquid is mostly absorbed before adding the next ladle. This process will take about 18-20 minutes, and the rice should become creamy but still have a slight bite.

5. **Add the vegetables:**

In the last 5 minutes of cooking, stir in the peas and chopped asparagus. Cook until the vegetables are tender.

6. **Finish with Parmesan and butter:**

Remove the risotto from heat, stir in the Parmesan cheese and butter. Season with salt and pepper to taste. If desired, add a bit of lemon zest for a bright finish.

7. **Serve:**

Garnish with fresh parsley or basil and extra Parmesan if desired.

29. Whole Wheat Veggie Pizza

The whole wheat crust increases fiber, while the diversity of vegetables provides vitamins and antioxidants.

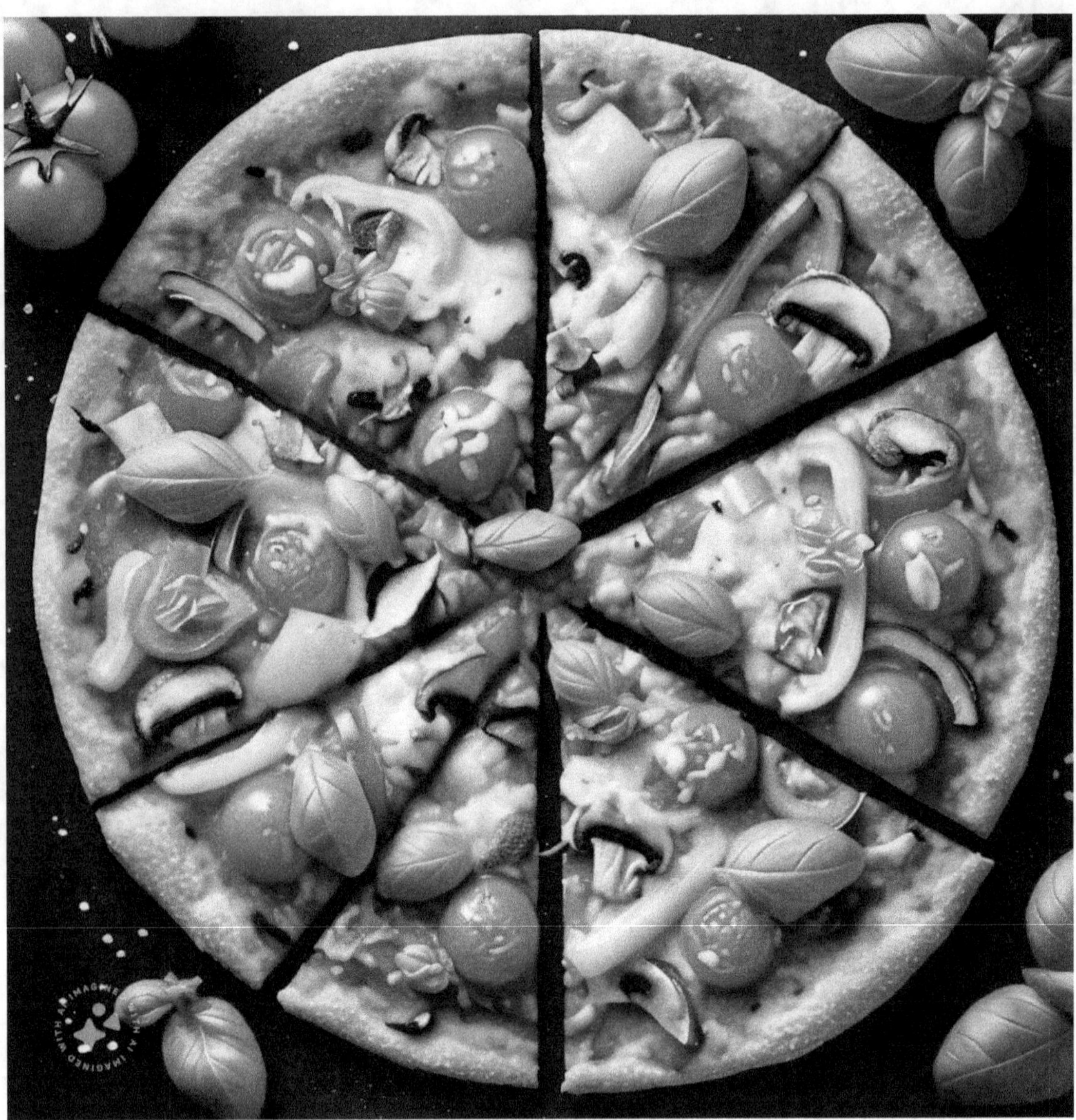

Ingredients:

For the dough:

- 2 ½ cups whole wheat flour

- 1 teaspoon active dry yeast

- 1 teaspoon sugar

- 1 teaspoon salt

- 1 tablespoon olive oil

- 1 cup warm water

For the toppings:

- 1/2 cup tomato sauce

- 1 ½ cups shredded mozzarella cheese

- 1/2 bell pepper, thinly sliced

- 1/2 red onion, thinly sliced

- 1/2 cup mushrooms, sliced

- 1/2 zucchini, thinly sliced

- 1/4 cup black olives, sliced

- 1 teaspoon dried oregano

- Fresh basil leaves, for garnish

- Olive oil, for drizzling

Instructions:

1. **Prepare the dough:**

In a small bowl, dissolve the yeast and sugar in warm water. Let it sit for 5-10 minutes until it becomes frothy. In a large mixing bowl, combine the whole wheat flour and salt.

Pour in the yeast mixture and olive oil. Mix until a dough forms, then knead on a floured surface for 5-7 minutes until smooth and elastic. Place the dough in an oiled bowl, cover, and let it rise for 1 hour.

2. **Preheat the oven:**

Set it to 220°C (425°F).

3. **Roll out the dough:**

After the dough has risen, punch it down and roll it out on a floured surface to form a pizza base. Transfer the dough to a baking sheet or pizza stone.

4. **Assemble the pizza:**

Spread the tomato sauce evenly over the pizza dough. Sprinkle the shredded mozzarella cheese on top.

Arrange the sliced bell peppers, onions, mushrooms, zucchini, and olives over the cheese. Sprinkle dried oregano over the veggies.

5. **Bake the pizza:**

Place the pizza in the preheated oven and bake for 12-15 minutes, or until the crust is golden and the cheese is melted and bubbly.

6. **Serve:**

Remove the pizza from the oven, drizzle with a little olive oil, and garnish with fresh basil leaves. Slice and serve hot.

30. Mediterranean Couscous Salad

This salad is high in fiber and plant-based proteins, which boost heart health and digestion.

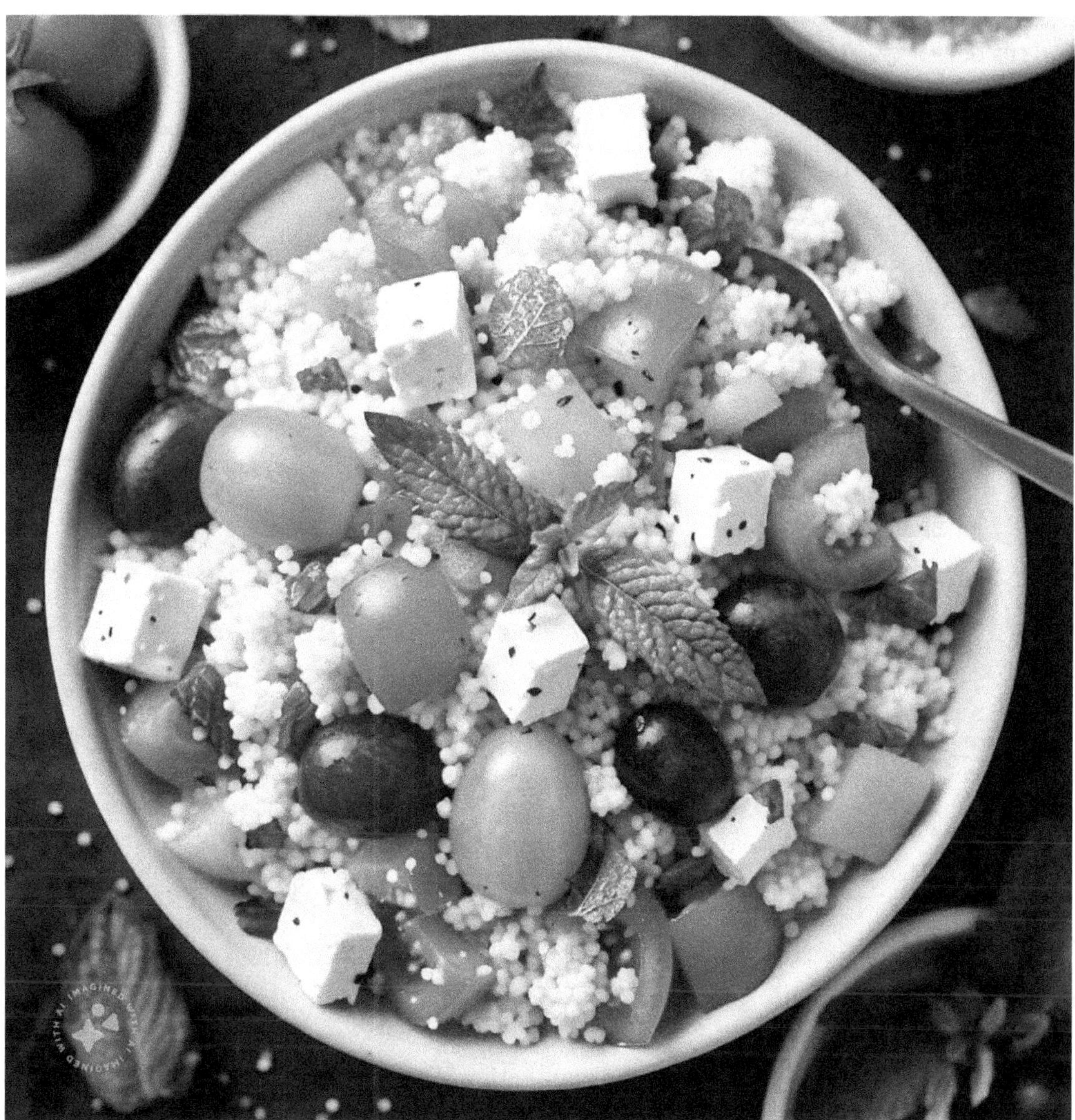

Ingredients:

- 1 cup couscous

- 1 ¼ cups boiling water

- 1 cup cherry tomatoes, halved

- 1 cucumber, diced

- 1/2 cup black olives, pitted and sliced

- 1/2 cup feta cheese, crumbled

- 1/4 red onion, finely chopped

- 1/4 cup fresh parsley, chopped

- 1/4 cup olive oil

- 2 tablespoons lemon juice

- 1 teaspoon dried oregano

- Salt and pepper, to taste

Instructions:

1. **Prepare the couscous:**

In a large bowl, combine the couscous and boiling water. Cover the bowl with a lid or plastic wrap and let it sit for about 5 minutes, or until the couscous absorbs the water. Fluff with a fork once done.

2. **Combine the ingredients:**

In a large mixing bowl, add the halved cherry tomatoes, diced cucumber, sliced olives, crumbled feta cheese, chopped red onion, and fresh parsley.

3. **Make the dressing:**

In a small bowl, whisk together the olive oil, lemon juice, dried oregano, salt, and pepper.

4. **Mix everything together:**

Add the fluffed couscous to the vegetable and feta mixture. Pour the dressing over the salad and toss gently until everything is well combined.

5. **Serve:**

Allow the salad to sit for about 10-15 minutes to let the flavors meld. Serve chilled or at room temperature.

31. Butternut Squash Soup

This creamy soup is low in calories but high in vitamins A and C, which promote immune and digestive health.

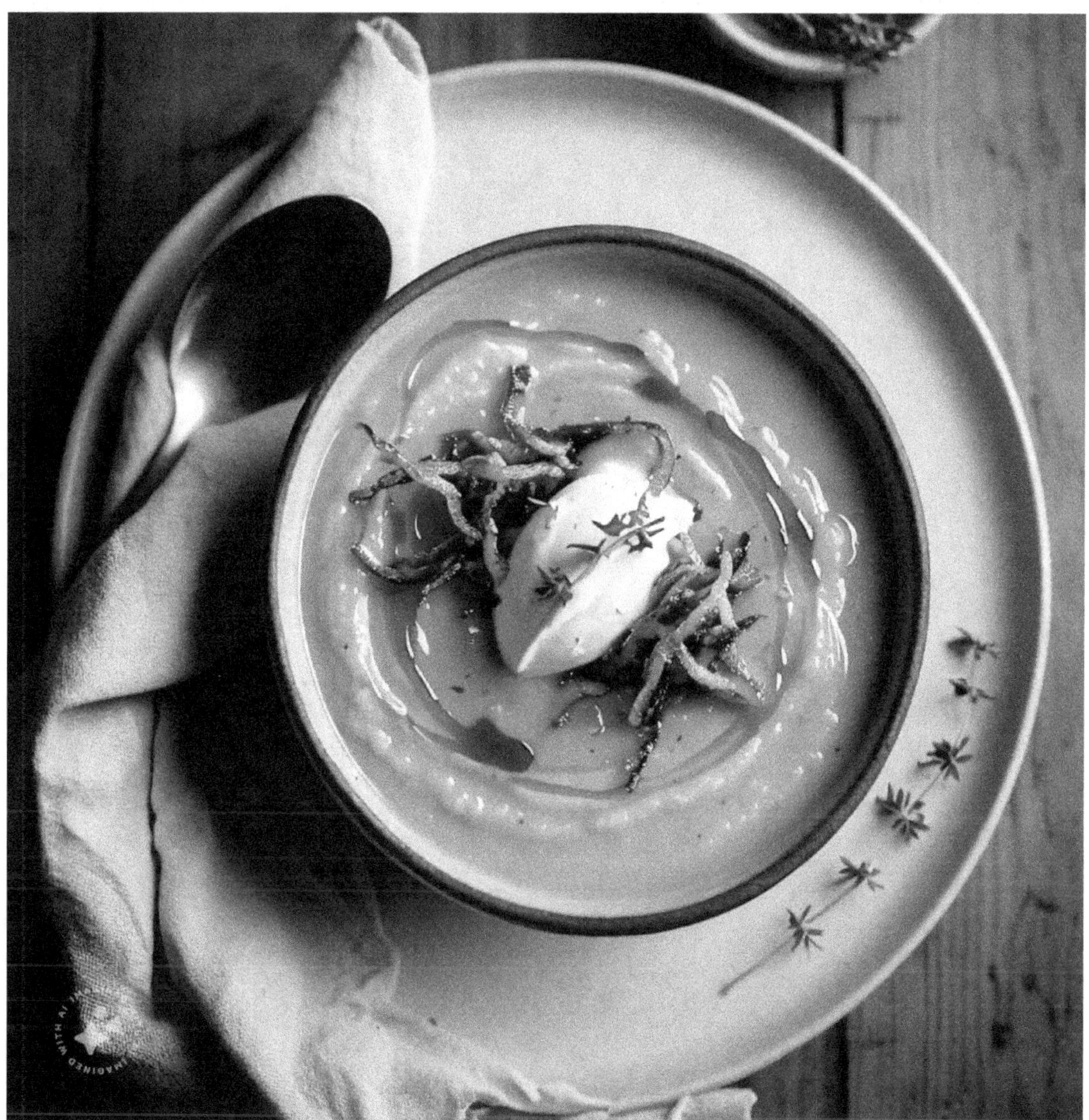

Ingredients:

- 1 medium butternut squash (about 1.5 kg), peeled and cubed

- 1 onion, chopped

- 2 cloves garlic, minced

- 3 cups vegetable broth

- 1 cup coconut milk or heavy cream

- 1 teaspoon olive oil

- 1/2 teaspoon ground nutmeg

- 1/2 teaspoon ground cinnamon

- Salt and pepper, to taste

- Fresh parsley or chives, for garnish

Instructions:

1. **Sauté the onion and garlic:**

In a large pot, heat olive oil over medium heat. Add the chopped onion and sauté for about 5 minutes until soft. Stir in the minced garlic and cook for another 1-2 minutes until fragrant.

2. **Cook the butternut squash:**

Add the cubed butternut squash to the pot, followed by the vegetable broth. Bring to a boil, then reduce the heat and simmer for about 20-25 minutes, or until the squash is tender.

3. **Blend the soup:**

Remove the pot from heat. Using an immersion blender, blend the soup until smooth. Alternatively, you can transfer the soup in batches to a countertop blender, blending until creamy.

4. **Add cream and seasonings:**

Return the blended soup to the pot (if using a countertop blender). Stir in the coconut milk or heavy cream, ground nutmeg, ground cinnamon, salt, and pepper. Heat the soup over low heat until warmed through.

5. **Serve:**

Ladle the soup into bowls and garnish with fresh parsley or chives.

32.   Whole Wheat Pita Bread with Hummus

Hummus, a high-fiber, nutrient-dense snack, provides healthy fats and protein, while whole wheat pita aids digestion.

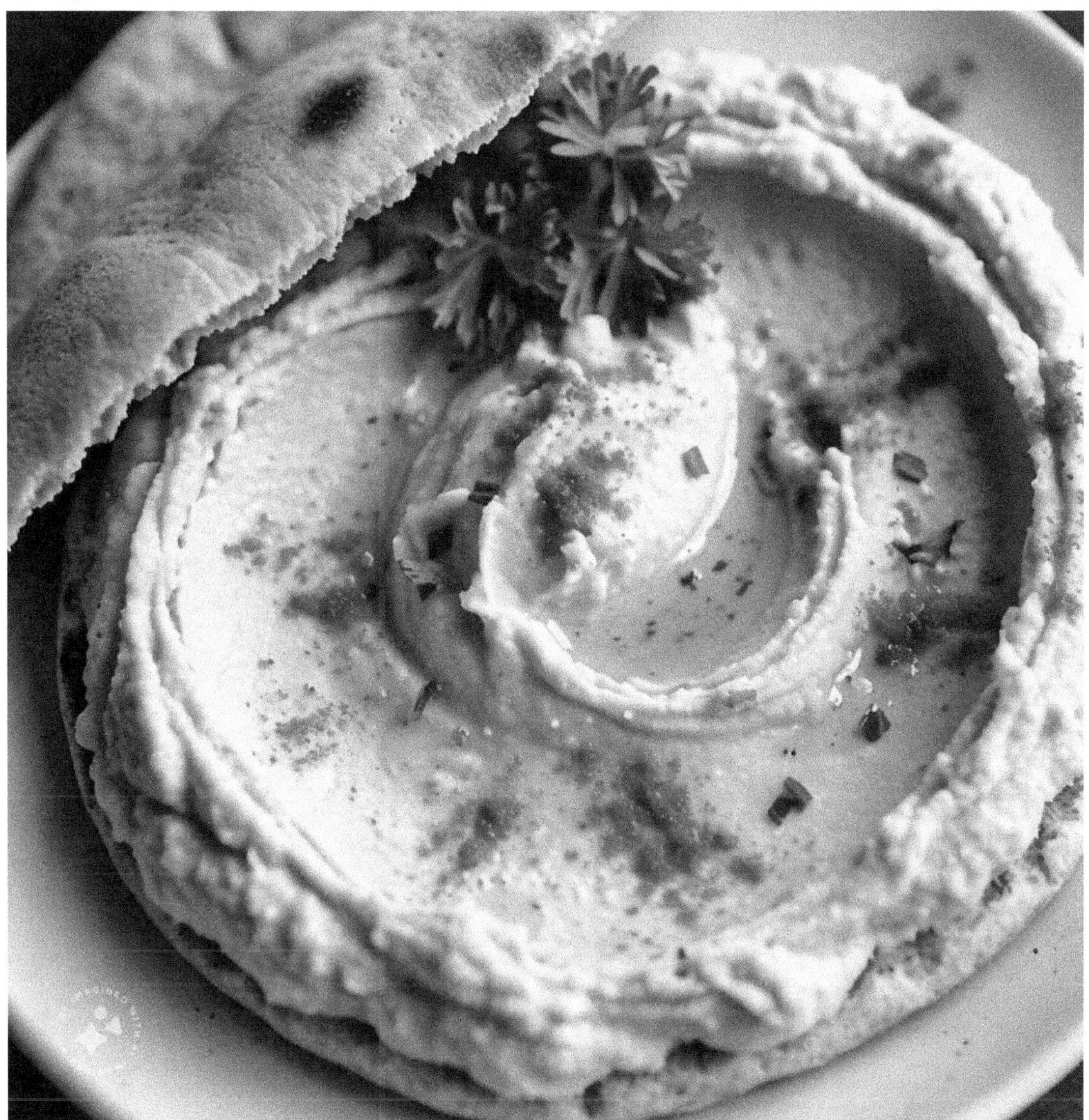

Whole Wheat Pita Bread Ingredients:

- 2 cups whole wheat flour

- 1 teaspoon active dry yeast

- 1 teaspoon sugar

- 1 teaspoon salt

- 1 tablespoon olive oil

- 3/4 cup warm water

Hummus Ingredients:

- 1 can (400g) chickpeas, drained and rinsed

- 2 tablespoons tahini

- 2 tablespoons olive oil

- 2 cloves garlic, minced

- 2 tablespoons lemon juice

- Salt, to taste

- Water (as needed for consistency)

- Paprika or olive oil (for garnish)

Instructions:

1. Activate the yeast:

In a small bowl, mix the warm water, sugar, and yeast. Let it sit for about 5-10 minutes until frothy.

2. Mix the dough:

In a large bowl, combine the whole wheat flour and salt. Make a well in the center and pour in the yeast mixture and olive oil. Mix until a dough forms.

3. Knead the dough:

Transfer the dough to a floured surface and knead for about 5-7 minutes until smooth and elastic.

4. Let it rise:

Place the dough in a lightly oiled bowl, cover with a damp cloth, and let it rise in a warm place for about 1 hour, or until doubled in size.

5. Shape the pitas:

Once risen, punch down the dough and divide it into 8 equal pieces. Roll each piece into a ball, then flatten into a circle about 1/4 inch thick.

6. Cook the pitas:

Preheat a skillet or baking stone over medium-high heat. Cook each pita for about 2-3 minutes on each side, or until puffed and lightly browned. Keep them warm in a towel.

Making the Hummus:

1. Blend the ingredients:

In a food processor, combine the chickpeas, tahini, olive oil, minced garlic, lemon juice, and salt. Blend until smooth.

2. Adjust the consistency:

If the hummus is too thick, add a little water, one tablespoon at a time, until you reach your desired consistency.

3. Serve:

Transfer the hummus to a serving bowl and drizzle with olive oil and sprinkle with paprika for garnish.

33. Chickpea and Spinach Stew

This substantial stew is high in fiber, iron, and plant-based proteins, which promote digestive and cardiovascular health.

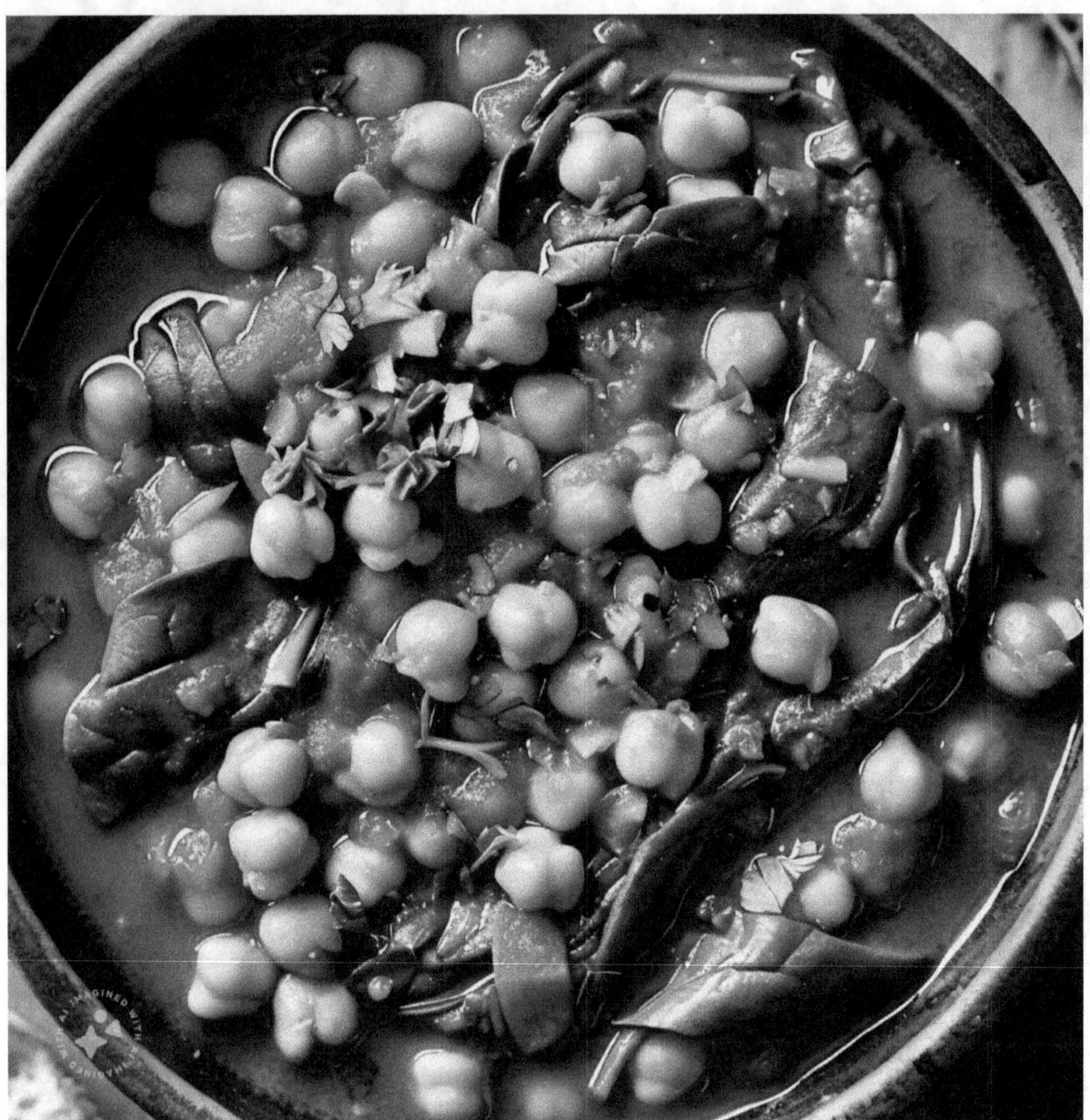

Ingredients:

- 1 can (400g) chickpeas, drained and rinsed

- 2 cups fresh spinach, chopped (or 1 cup frozen spinach)

- 1 can (400g) diced tomatoes

- 1 onion, chopped

- 3 cloves garlic, minced

- 1 teaspoon ground cumin

- 1 teaspoon paprika

- 1/2 teaspoon turmeric

- 2 tablespoons olive oil

- 1 cup vegetable broth or water

- Salt and pepper, to taste

- Fresh parsley or cilantro, for garnish

- Lemon wedges (for serving)

Instructions:

1. **Sauté the aromatics:**

In a large pot, heat the olive oil over medium heat. Add the chopped onion and cook for about 5 minutes, or until softened. Stir in the minced garlic and cook for an additional 1-2 minutes until fragrant.

2. **Add the spices:**

Sprinkle in the cumin, paprika, and turmeric, stirring to coat the onions and garlic. Cook for about 1 minute to release the flavors.

3. **Combine the ingredients:**

Add the diced tomatoes (with their juice) and vegetable broth. Stir to combine, then bring the mixture to a simmer.

4. **Add the chickpeas:**

Stir in the drained chickpeas and season with salt and pepper. Allow the stew to simmer for about 10-15 minutes, stirring occasionally, until it thickens slightly.

5. Incorporate the spinach:

Add the chopped fresh spinach and cook for an additional 5 minutes until wilted. If using frozen spinach, stir it in and cook until heated through.

6. Serve:

Remove from heat and taste for seasoning, adjusting salt and pepper as needed. Garnish with fresh parsley or cilantro and serve with lemon wedges on the side.

34. Stuffed Zucchini Boats

Zucchini is minimal in carbs and calories, and the filling makes for a protein-rich, fulfilling lunch.

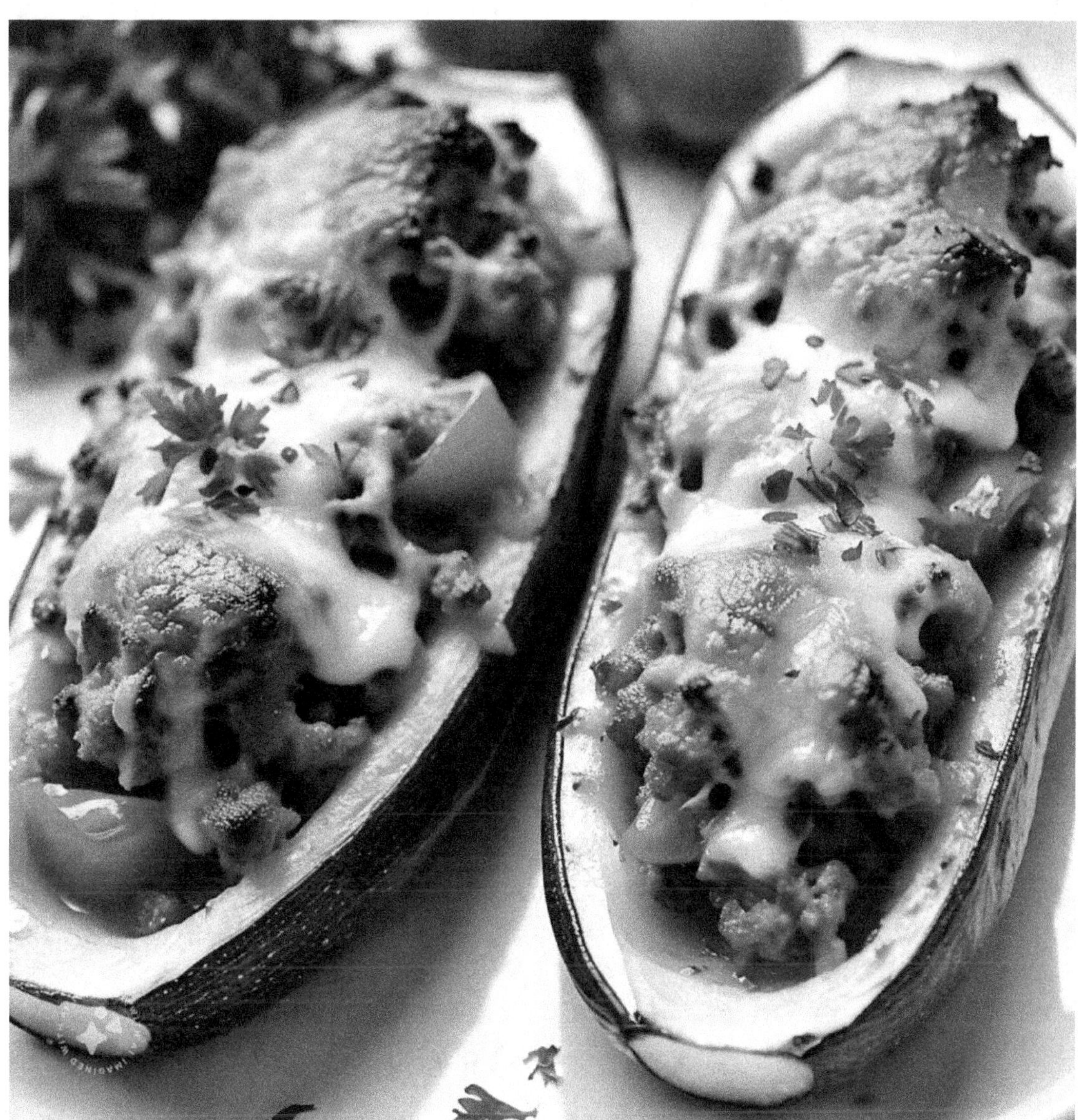

Ingredients:

- 4 medium zucchinis

- 1 cup cooked quinoa

- 1 cup cherry tomatoes, halved

- 1/2 cup mozzarella cheese, shredded

- 1/4 cup fresh basil, chopped (plus extra for garnish)

- 1 tablespoon olive oil

- 2 cloves garlic, minced

- 1/2 teaspoon dried oregano

- Salt and pepper, to taste

- Grated Parmesan cheese (optional, for topping)

Instructions:

1. **Preheat the oven:**

Set it to 190°C (375°F).

2. **Prepare the zucchinis:**

Cut the zucchinis in half lengthwise and scoop out the seeds with a spoon to create boats. Place them cut-side up in a baking dish.

3. **Cook the filling:**

In a large skillet, heat olive oil over medium heat. Add minced garlic and sauté for 1-2 minutes until fragrant. Stir in the halved cherry tomatoes and cook for another 3-4 minutes until they start to soften.

4. **Combine ingredients:**

In a large bowl, mix the cooked quinoa, sautéed tomatoes, shredded mozzarella, chopped basil, dried oregano, salt, and pepper.

5. **Stuff the zucchinis:**

Spoon the quinoa mixture into each zucchini boat, pressing down gently to pack it in. If desired, sprinkle additional mozzarella or grated Parmesan cheese on top.

6. **Bake the zucchini boats:**

Place the baking dish in the preheated oven and bake for 20-25 minutes, or until the zucchinis are tender and the cheese is melted and bubbly.

7. **Serve:**

Remove from the oven and let cool slightly. Garnish with extra fresh basil before serving.

35.   Oatmeal with Berries

A fiber-rich breakfast that regulates blood sugar, and the berries include antioxidants that promote overall health.

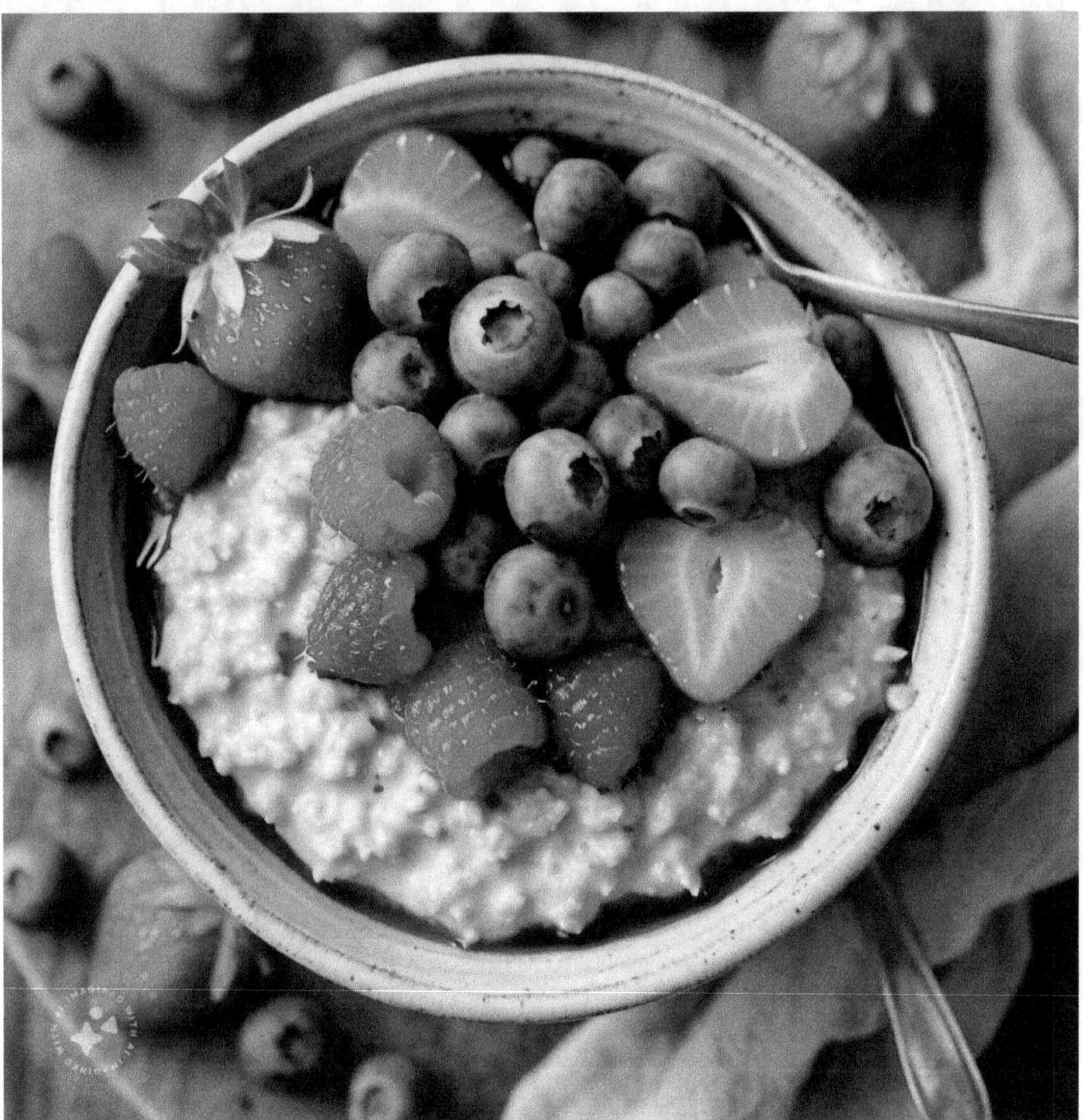

Ingredients:

- 1 cup rolled oats

- 2 cups almond milk (or any milk of your choice)

- 1/2 tsp vanilla extract (optional)

- 1 tbsp honey or maple syrup (optional)

- A pinch of salt

- Fresh berries (such as blueberries, raspberries, strawberries)

- Chopped nuts, seeds, or coconut flakes for topping (optional)

Instructions:

1. **Cook the Oats:**

   - In a medium saucepan, combine the rolled oats, almond milk, and a pinch of salt. Bring the mixture to a boil over medium heat.

   - Reduce the heat to low and simmer for 5-7 minutes, stirring occasionally, until the oats are soft and have absorbed most of the liquid.

2. **Add Flavor:**

   - If desired, stir in the vanilla extract and sweetener (honey or maple syrup) once the oats are cooked.

3. **Serve:**

   - Pour the oatmeal into a bowl. Top it with fresh berries of your choice.

   - Sprinkle with additional toppings like chopped nuts, seeds, or coconut flakes for added texture and flavor.

4. **Enjoy:**

   - Serve warm and enjoy your healthy, nutritious breakfast!

36. Vegetarian Chili

This chili is high in plant-based proteins and fiber, which will keep you satisfied while also benefiting your heart and digestion.

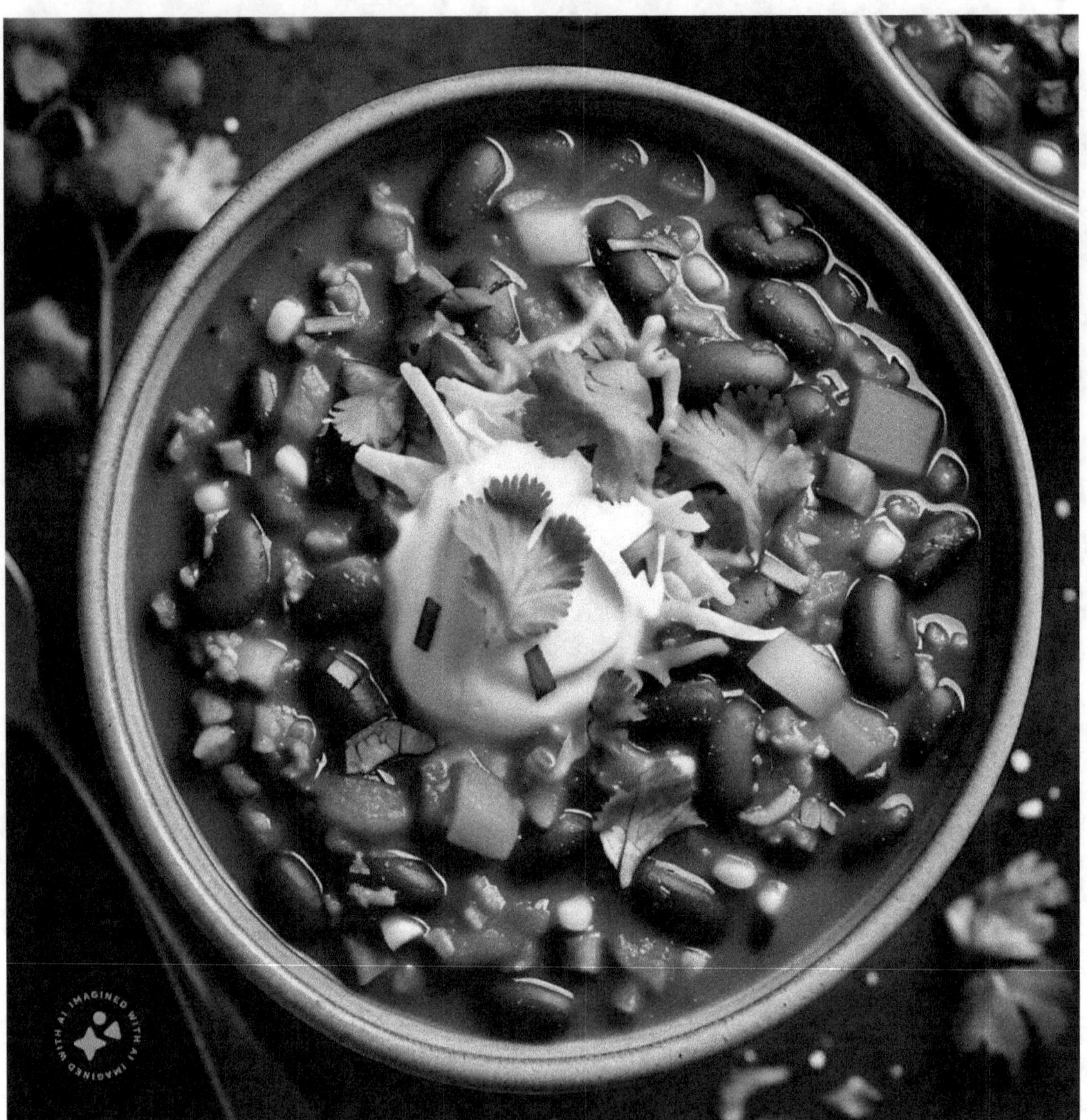

Ingredients:

- 1 tbsp olive oil

- 1 onion, diced

- 2 cloves garlic, minced

- 1 bell pepper, diced (any color)

- 1 zucchini, diced

- 1 carrot, diced

- 1 can (15 oz) black beans, drained and rinsed

- 1 can (15 oz) kidney beans, drained and rinsed

- 1 can (15 oz) diced tomatoes

- 1 can (8 oz) tomato sauce

- 1 cup vegetable broth

- 2 tbsp chili powder

- 1 tsp cumin

- 1/2 tsp smoked paprika

- 1/2 tsp ground cayenne pepper (optional, for extra heat)

- Salt and pepper to taste

- Fresh cilantro for garnish (optional)

- Sour cream or avocado for topping (optional)

Instructions:

1. **Sauté Vegetables:**

   - Heat olive oil in a large pot over medium heat. Add the diced onion, garlic, and bell pepper. Sauté for about 5 minutes until the vegetables start to soften.

   - Add the diced zucchini and carrot, and cook for another 5 minutes, stirring occasionally.

2. **Add Spices:**

   - Stir in the chili powder, cumin, smoked paprika, and cayenne pepper (if using). Cook for 1-2 minutes until the spices are fragrant.

3. **Add Beans and Tomatoes:**

   - Add the black beans, kidney beans, diced tomatoes (with their juice), tomato sauce, and vegetable broth. Stir to combine.

4. **Simmer:**

   - Bring the mixture to a boil, then reduce the heat to low. Cover and simmer for 20-30 minutes, allowing the flavors to meld together. Stir occasionally.

5. **Season:**

   - Taste the chili and season with salt and pepper as needed. Adjust the spices if you want more heat.

6. **Serve:**

   - Ladle the chili into bowls. Garnish with fresh cilantro, and top with sour cream or avocado if desired.

37. Bulgur Wheat Tabbouleh

A high-fiber, low-fat dish that aids digestion and contains critical vitamins from fresh herbs and vegetables.

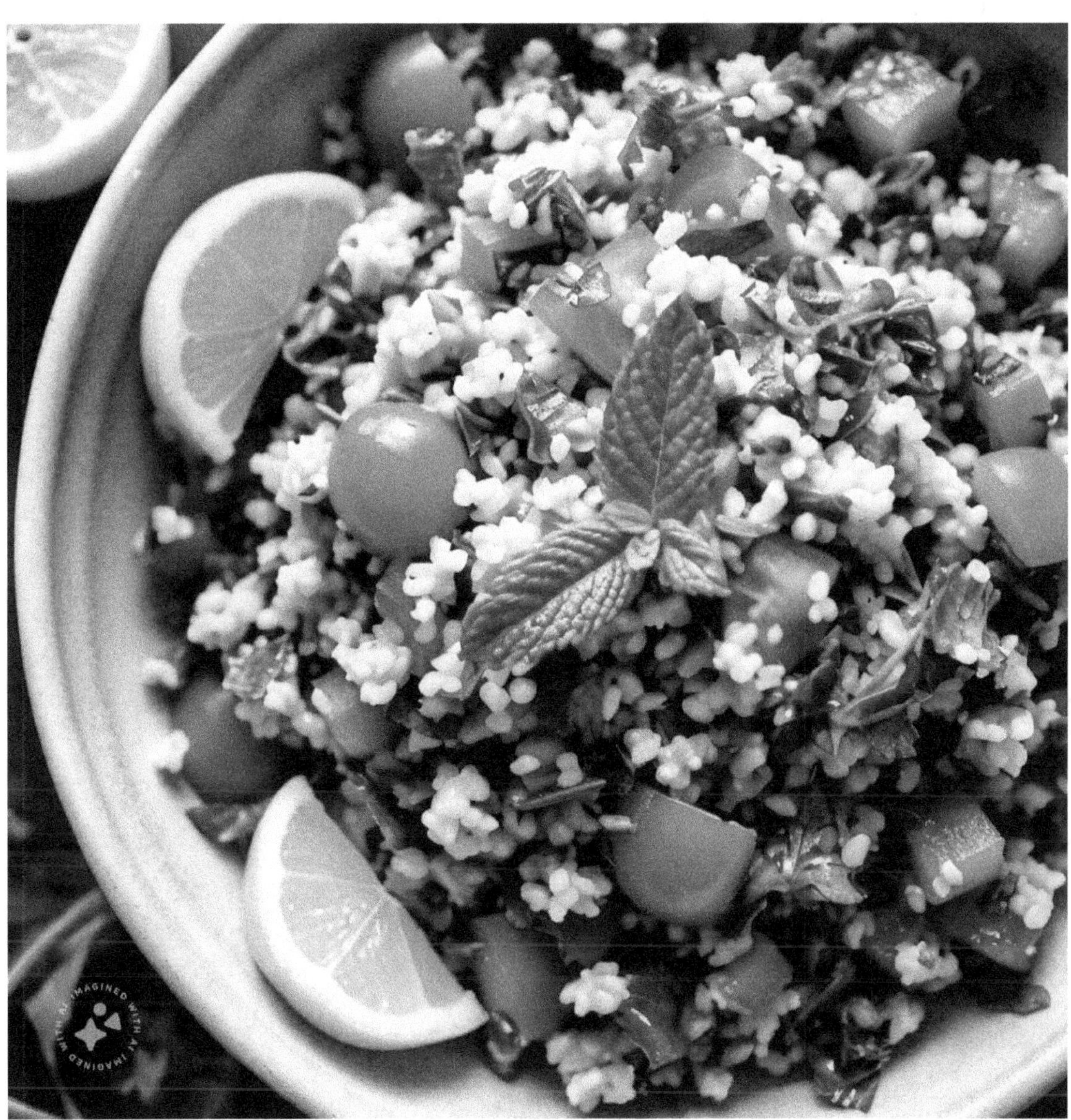

Ingredients:

- 1 cup bulgur wheat

- 1 1/2 cups boiling water

- 1 bunch fresh parsley, finely chopped (about 2 cups)

- 1/2 bunch fresh mint, finely chopped (about 1/2 cup)

- 3-4 tomatoes, finely diced

- 1 small cucumber, finely diced (optional)

- 4-5 green onions, finely chopped

- 1/4 cup olive oil

- Juice of 2 lemons (about 1/4 cup)

- Salt and pepper to taste

Instructions:

1. **Prepare the Bulgur:**

   - Place the bulgur wheat in a large bowl. Pour the boiling water over the bulgur, cover the bowl with a plate or lid, and let it sit for 15-20 minutes until the bulgur has absorbed the water and softened.

   - Once the bulgur is ready, fluff it with a fork to separate the grains.

2. **Chop Vegetables and Herbs:**

   - While the bulgur is soaking, finely chop the parsley, mint, tomatoes, cucumber (if using), and green onions.

3. **Combine Ingredients:**

   - Add the chopped parsley, mint, tomatoes, cucumber, and green onions to the bulgur. Mix everything together.

4. **Add Dressing:**

   - In a small bowl, whisk together the olive oil and lemon juice. Pour the dressing over the tabbouleh and toss well to coat all the ingredients.

5. **Season:**

   - Season the tabbouleh with salt and pepper to taste. Adjust the lemon juice and olive oil if needed, based on your preference.

6. **Serve:**

   - Let the tabbouleh sit for about 30 minutes before serving to allow the flavors to meld. Serve chilled or at room temperature.

38. Baked Falafel Wraps

Falafel contains plant-based protein, and baking minimizes fat levels, making it a healthy and tasty option.

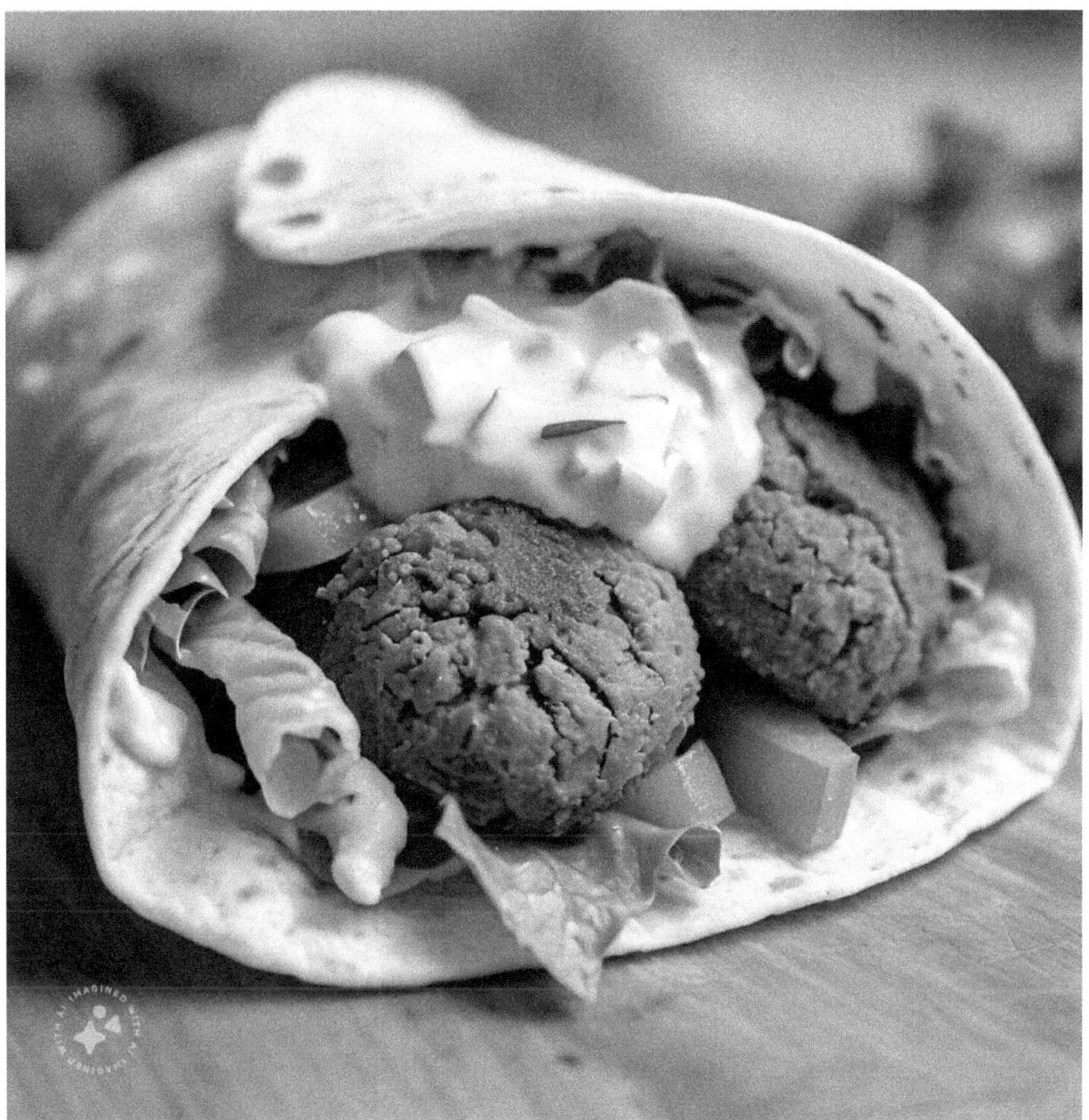

Ingredients:

For the Baked Falafel:

- 1 can (15 oz) chickpeas, drained and rinsed

- 1 small onion, roughly chopped

- 2 cloves garlic, minced

- 1/4 cup fresh parsley

- 1/4 cup fresh cilantro (optional)

- 1 tsp ground cumin

- 1 tsp ground coriander

- 1/2 tsp ground paprika

- 1/4 tsp baking powder

- 2 tbsp flour (or chickpea flour)

- Salt and pepper to taste

- 1-2 tbsp olive oil for brushing

For the Wraps:

- 4 large wraps or pita bread

- Lettuce, chopped

- 1-2 tomatoes, sliced

- 1 small cucumber, sliced (optional)

- Red onion, thinly sliced (optional)

- Tzatziki sauce (store-bought or homemade, see below)

For Homemade Tzatziki:

- 1 cup Greek yogurt

- 1/2 cucumber, grated and drained

- 1 clove garlic, minced

- 1 tbsp olive oil

- Juice of 1/2 lemon

- 1 tbsp fresh dill or mint (optional)

- Salt and pepper to taste

Instructions:

1. Preheat Oven:

   - Preheat your oven to 375°F (190°C) and line a baking sheet with parchment paper or lightly grease it.

2. Prepare the Falafel Mixture:

   - In a food processor, combine the chickpeas, onion, garlic, parsley, cilantro (if using), cumin, coriander, paprika, baking powder, flour, salt, and pepper. Pulse until the mixture is combined but still slightly chunky, not fully smooth.

   - If the mixture is too wet, add a little more flour to achieve a moldable consistency.

3. Shape and Bake the Falafel:

   - Form the falafel mixture into small balls or patties, about 1 1/2 inches in diameter, and place them on the prepared baking sheet.

   - Lightly brush the tops with olive oil to help them brown.

   - Bake for 20-25 minutes, flipping halfway through, until the falafel is golden and crispy on the outside.

4. Make the Tzatziki Sauce (optional):

   - In a small bowl, combine the Greek yogurt, grated cucumber (make sure to squeeze out the excess water), garlic, olive oil, lemon juice, fresh dill or mint (if using), salt, and pepper. Stir well to combine.

5. **Assemble the Wraps:**

   - Warm the wraps or pita bread slightly, if desired.

   - Spread a generous amount of tzatziki sauce on each wrap, then top with baked falafel, lettuce, tomato slices, cucumber, and red onion.

6. **Serve:**

   - Wrap tightly and serve immediately. You can also serve with extra tzatziki sauce on the side.

39. Mushroom and Spinach Risotto

This creamy recipe is high in fiber and antioxidants, which promote heart health and intestinal wellness.

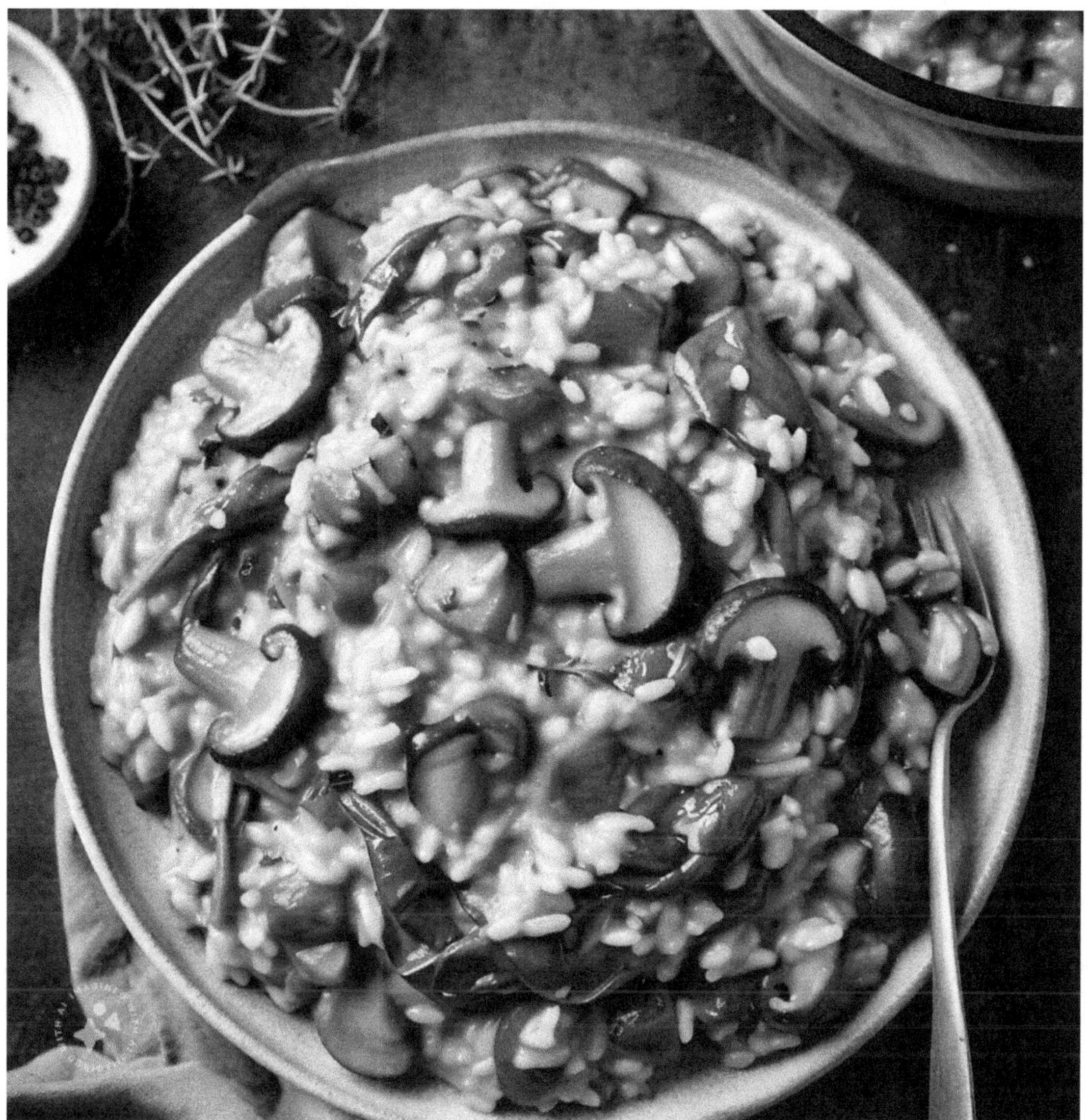

Ingredients:

- 1 1/2 cups arborio rice

- 1 tbsp olive oil

- 2 tbsp butter

- 1 onion, finely chopped

- 3 cloves garlic, minced

- 1 1/2 cups mushrooms, sliced (cremini, button, or your choice)

- 1/2 cup white wine (optional)

- 4-5 cups vegetable broth, kept warm

- 2 cups fresh spinach, roughly chopped

- 1/2 cup grated Parmesan cheese (plus extra for serving)

- Salt and pepper to taste

- Fresh parsley for garnish (optional)

Instructions:

1. **Sauté Mushrooms:**

   - Heat 1 tablespoon of olive oil and 1 tablespoon of butter in a large pan over medium heat.

   - Add the sliced mushrooms and cook for 5-7 minutes until browned and soft. Remove the mushrooms from the pan and set aside.

2. **Sauté Onion and Garlic:**

   - In the same pan, melt the remaining 1 tablespoon of butter. Add the chopped onion and cook for about 3-4 minutes until softened and translucent.

   - Stir in the minced garlic and cook for 1 more minute until fragrant.

3. **Add the Arborio Rice:**

   - Add the arborio rice to the pan and stir for 2-3 minutes, allowing the rice to lightly toast.

4. **Deglaze with Wine (Optional):**

   - If using, pour in the white wine and stir until the wine is mostly absorbed by the rice.

5. **Cook the Risotto:**

   - Begin adding the warm vegetable broth, one ladleful at a time, stirring frequently. Allow the liquid to absorb before adding the next ladleful of broth.

   - Continue adding broth and stirring for about 18-20 minutes, until the rice is creamy and tender but still slightly firm (al dente).

6. **Add Mushrooms and Spinach:**

   - Stir the sautéed mushrooms and chopped spinach into the risotto. Continue to cook for 2-3 minutes until the spinach wilts.

7. **Add Parmesan:**

   - Stir in the grated Parmesan cheese and season with salt and pepper to taste.

8. **Serve:**

   - Serve the risotto hot, garnished with extra Parmesan cheese and fresh parsley, if desired.

40. Lentil and Sweet Potato Curry

This curry, which is high in fiber, plant-based protein, and vitamins, is both nutritious and beneficial to blood sugar regulation.

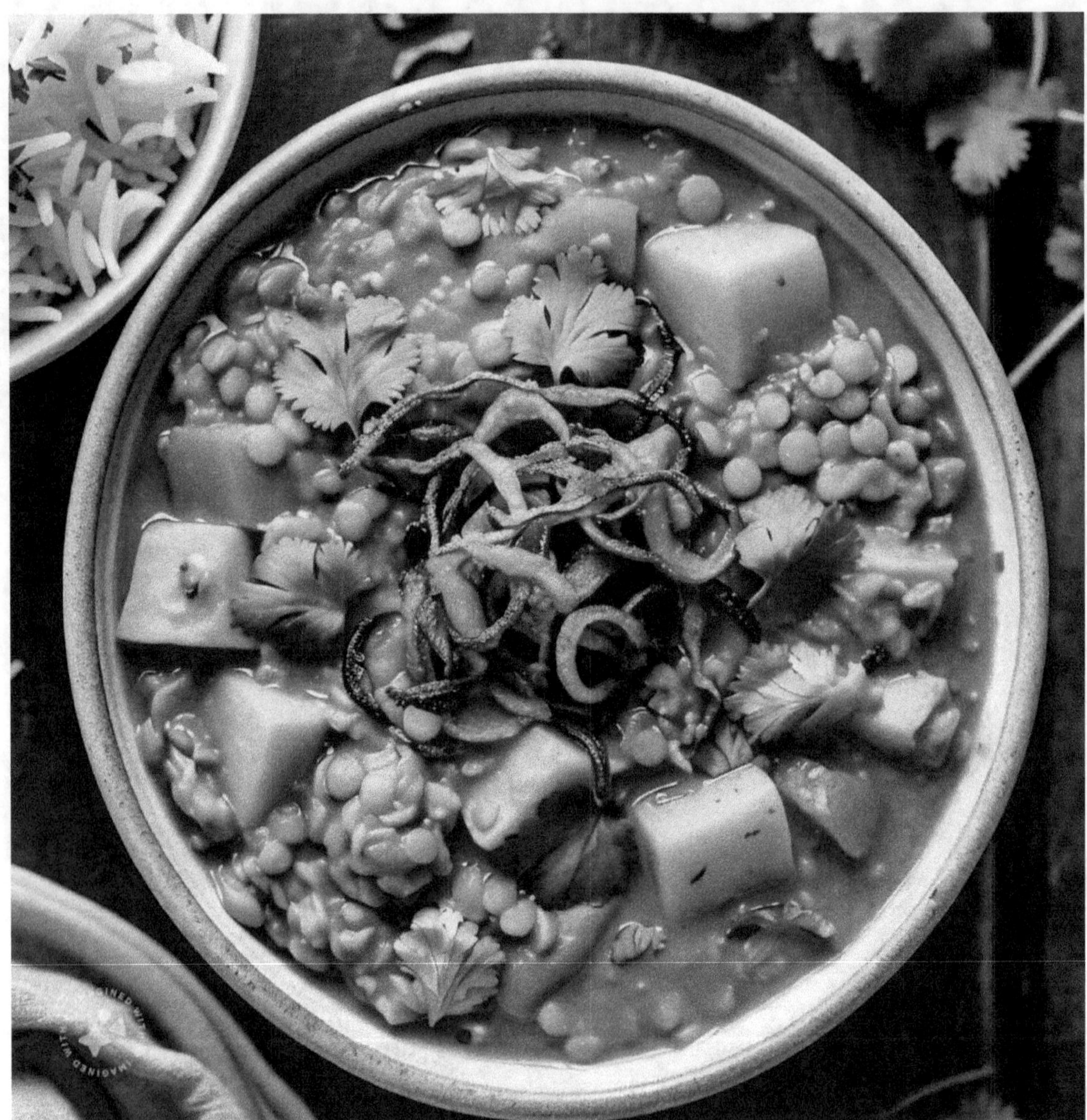

Ingredients:

- 1 tbsp olive oil or coconut oil

- 1 onion, diced

- 3 cloves garlic, minced

- 1 tbsp fresh ginger, minced

- 1 tbsp curry powder

- 1 tsp ground cumin

- 1/2 tsp ground turmeric

- 1/2 tsp ground coriander

- 1/4 tsp chili flakes or cayenne pepper (optional, for heat)

- 1 1/2 cups dried lentils (red or green), rinsed

- 2 medium sweet potatoes, peeled and diced

- 1 can (14 oz) coconut milk

- 3 cups vegetable broth (or water)

- 1 can (14 oz) diced tomatoes

- Salt and pepper to taste

- Fresh cilantro for garnish (optional)

- Lime wedges for serving (optional)

Instructions:

1. **Sauté the Vegetables:**

   - Heat the olive oil in a large pot over medium heat. Add the diced onion and cook for 4-5 minutes until softened.

   - Stir in the minced garlic and ginger, and cook for another 1-2 minutes until fragrant.

2. **Add the Spices:**

   - Add the curry powder, cumin, turmeric, coriander, and chili flakes (if using). Stir to coat the onions and cook for about 1 minute to release the flavors of the spices.

3. **Add Lentils and Sweet Potatoes:**

   - Add the rinsed lentils and diced sweet potatoes to the pot. Stir to combine with the onion and spice mixture.

4. **Pour in Liquids:**

   - Add the coconut milk, vegetable broth, and diced tomatoes (with their juices). Stir well to combine all the ingredients.

5. **Simmer:**

   - Bring the mixture to a boil, then reduce the heat to low. Cover the pot and let the curry simmer for 25-30 minutes, stirring occasionally, until the lentils and sweet potatoes are tender.

6. **Season and Adjust:**

   - Taste the curry and season with salt and pepper as needed. If the curry is too thick, you can add more vegetable broth to reach your desired consistency.

7. **Serve:**

   - Serve the curry over rice or with naan bread. Garnish with fresh cilantro and serve with lime wedges for a tangy finish, if desired.

41. Grilled Veggie Skewers

A colorful assortment of vegetables high in vitamins, fiber, and antioxidants, grilled to perfection for a nutritious lunch.

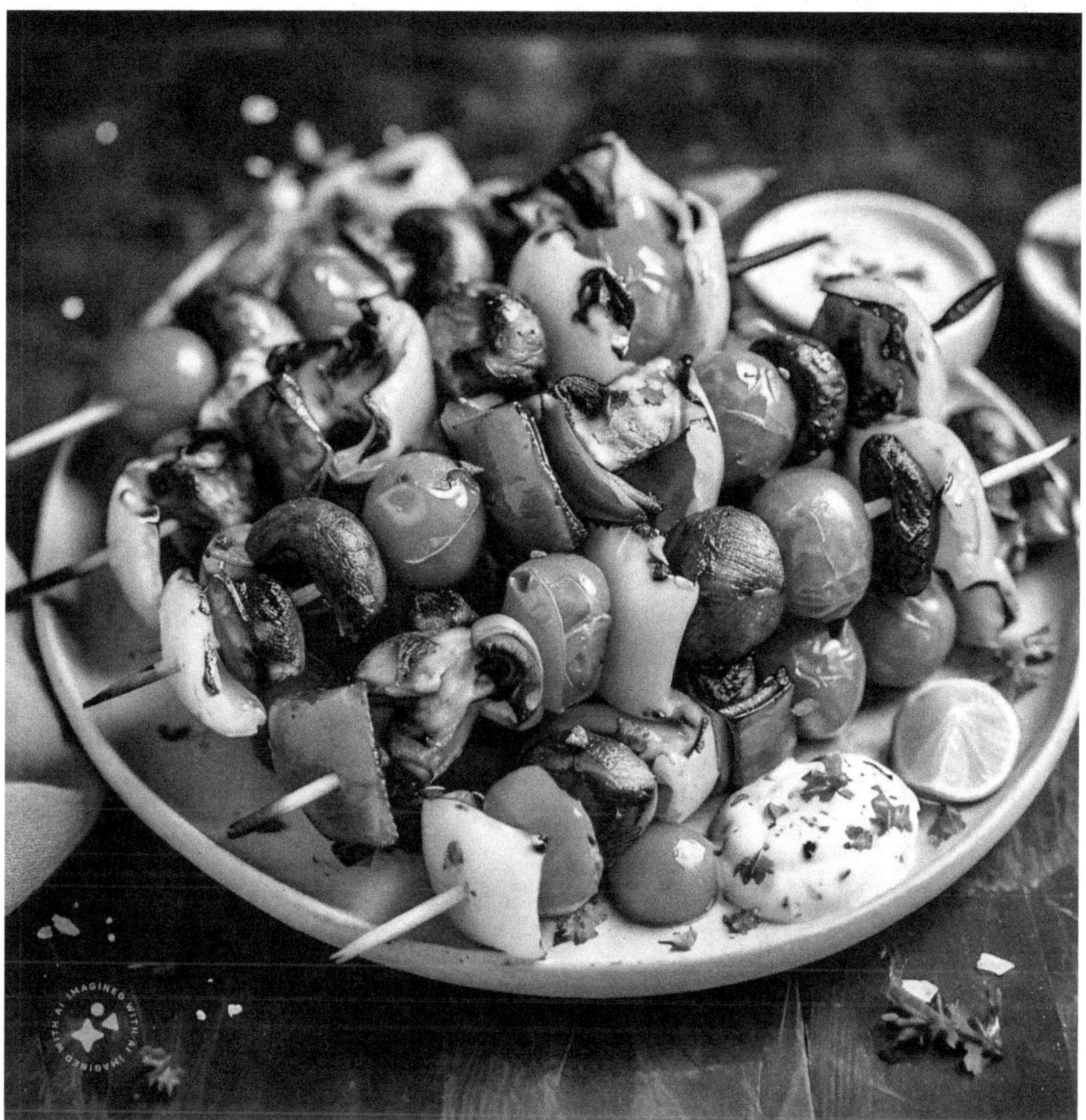

Ingredients:

- 2 zucchini, sliced into rounds or half-moons

- 2 bell peppers (red, yellow, or green), cut into 1-inch pieces

- 1 1/2 cups mushrooms (button, cremini, or portobello), stems removed

- 1 red onion, cut into chunks (optional)

- 2 tbsp olive oil

- 1 tbsp balsamic vinegar

- 2 cloves garlic, minced

- 1 tsp dried oregano

- 1 tsp dried thyme or rosemary

- Salt and pepper to taste

- Wooden or metal skewers

Instructions:

1. **Prepare the Skewers:**

   - If using wooden skewers, soak them in water for at least 30 minutes to prevent burning on the grill.

2. **Prepare the Vegetables:**

   - In a large bowl, combine the zucchini, bell peppers, mushrooms, and red onion (if using).

   - In a small bowl, whisk together the olive oil, balsamic vinegar, minced garlic, oregano, thyme, salt, and pepper.

   - Pour the marinade over the vegetables and toss well to coat. Let the vegetables marinate for 15-30 minutes for extra flavor.

3. **Assemble the Skewers:**

   - Thread the marinated vegetables onto the skewers, alternating between zucchini, peppers, mushrooms, and onions to create colorful skewers.

4. **Grill the Skewers:**

   - Preheat the grill to medium-high heat. Lightly oil the grill grates to prevent sticking.

   - Place the veggie skewers on the grill and cook for about 10-12 minutes, turning occasionally, until the vegetables are tender and slightly charred on the edges.

5. Serve:

   - Remove the skewers from the grill and serve immediately. These veggie skewers pair well with couscous, quinoa, or grilled proteins.

42. Caprese Salad

Fresh tomatoes and mozzarella are a delightful source of vitamins and good fats that promote skin and heart health.

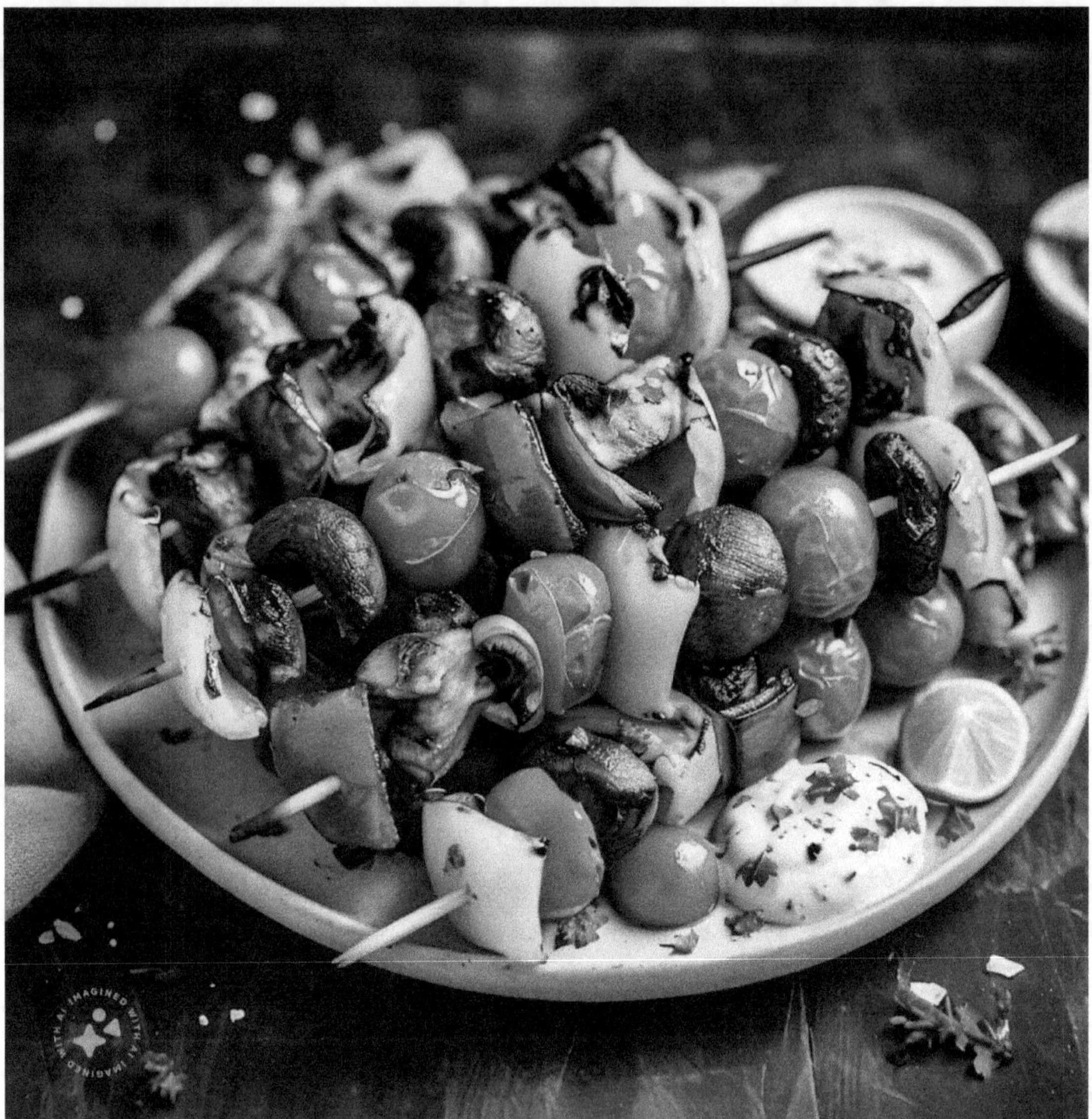

Ingredients:

- 3-4 ripe tomatoes, sliced (heirloom or vine-ripened for best flavor)

- 8 oz fresh mozzarella, sliced

- 1 bunch fresh basil leaves

- 2 tbsp extra virgin olive oil

- 1-2 tbsp balsamic glaze (store-bought or homemade)

- Salt and freshly ground black pepper, to taste

Instructions:

1. **Assemble the Salad:**

   - On a large platter or individual plates, alternate slices of tomato and fresh mozzarella, slightly overlapping them. Tuck basil leaves in between each layer of tomato and mozzarella.

2. **Drizzle with Olive Oil:**

   - Drizzle the extra virgin olive oil evenly over the tomatoes, mozzarella, and basil.

3. **Add Balsamic Glaze:**

   - Drizzle balsamic glaze over the top of the salad for a touch of sweetness and tang.

4. **Season:**

   - Sprinkle the salad with a pinch of salt and freshly ground black pepper to taste.

5. **Serve:**

   - Serve immediately, as a light appetizer or side dish.

.

43. Eggplant Parmesan

The eggplant is high in fibre and antioxidants, and the cheese provides calcium and protein for a well-balanced, tasty lunch.

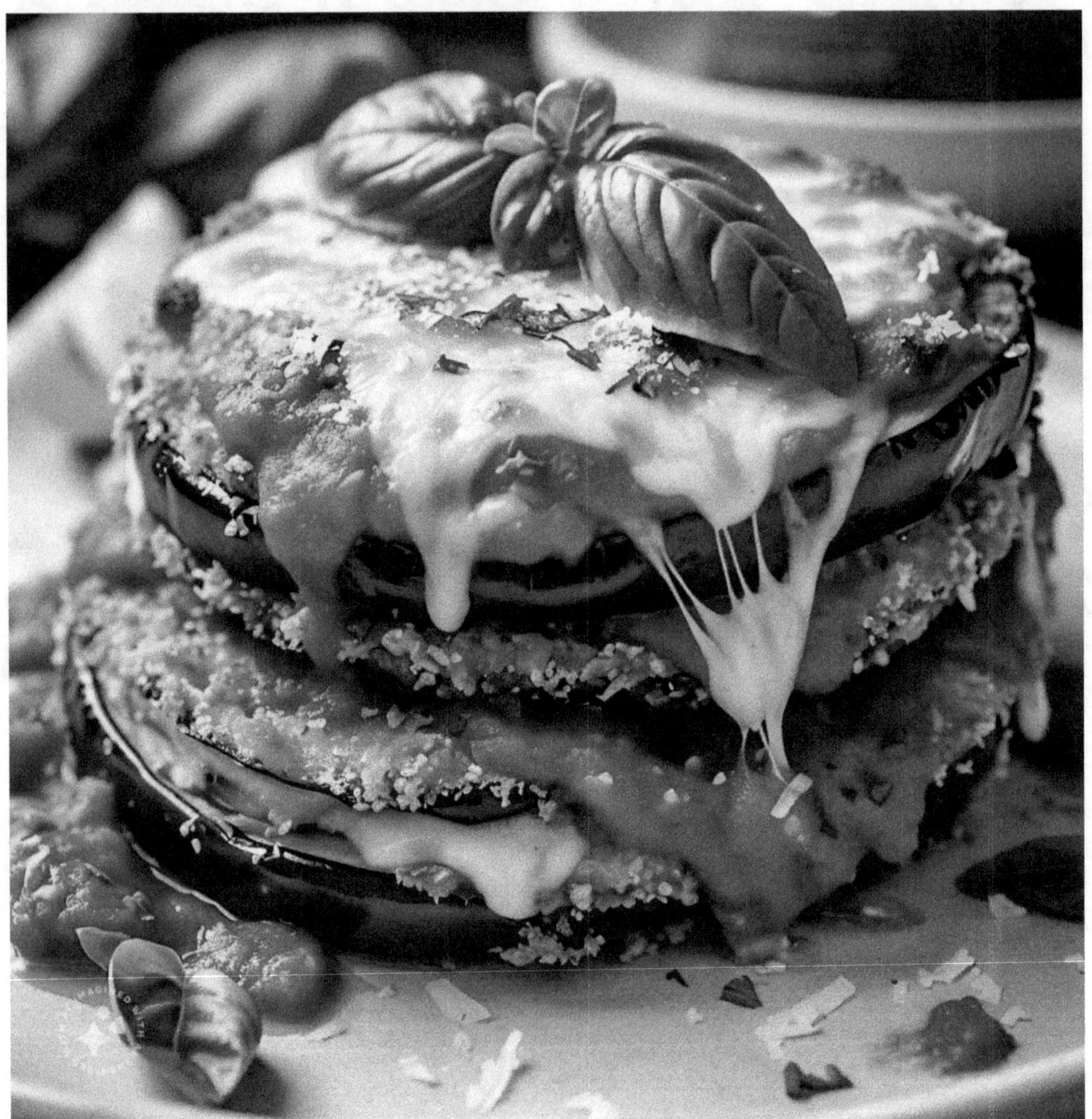

Ingredients:

- 2 large eggplants, sliced into 1/4-inch rounds

- 1 tsp salt (for prepping eggplant)

- 1 cup all-purpose flour

- 3 large eggs, beaten

- 1 1/2 cups breadcrumbs (Italian-style or Panko)

- 1/2 cup grated Parmesan cheese (plus extra for topping)

- 2 cups marinara sauce (store-bought or homemade)

- 2 cups shredded mozzarella cheese

- 2 tbsp olive oil (for greasing baking sheets)

- Fresh basil leaves for garnish (optional)

Instructions:

1. **Preheat the Oven:**

   - Preheat your oven to 400°F (200°C). Lightly grease two baking sheets with olive oil.

2. **Prepare the Eggplant:**

   - Lay the eggplant slices on paper towels and sprinkle them with salt on both sides. Let them sit for about 20-30 minutes to draw out excess moisture and bitterness. Afterward, pat them dry with paper towels.

3. **Coat the Eggplant:**

   - Set up a breading station with three shallow bowls. In the first bowl, place the flour. In the second bowl, beat the eggs. In the third bowl, combine the breadcrumbs and 1/2 cup of grated Parmesan.

   - Dredge each eggplant slice in the flour, dip it into the beaten eggs, and coat it with the breadcrumb mixture.

4. **Bake the Eggplant:**

   - Arrange the breaded eggplant slices in a single layer on the prepared baking sheets. Bake for 20-25 minutes, flipping halfway through, until the eggplant is golden and crispy.

5. **Assemble the Dish:**

   - Spread 1/2 cup of marinara sauce on the bottom of a large baking dish. Arrange a layer of baked eggplant slices over the sauce. Top with more marinara sauce,

then sprinkle with mozzarella and a bit of Parmesan cheese. Repeat the layers until all the eggplant is used, finishing with marinara and a final sprinkle of mozzarella and Parmesan.

6. **Bake the Eggplant Parmesan:**

   - Reduce the oven temperature to 375°F (190°C). Bake the assembled dish for 20-25 minutes, or until the cheese is melted and bubbly.

7. **Serve:**

   - Remove the dish from the oven and let it rest for a few minutes. Garnish with fresh basil leaves and extra Parmesan cheese, if desired.

44. Vegetable Stir Fry

A quick, nutrient-dense lunch with of vitamins, fiber, and antioxidants that promotes general health and digestion.

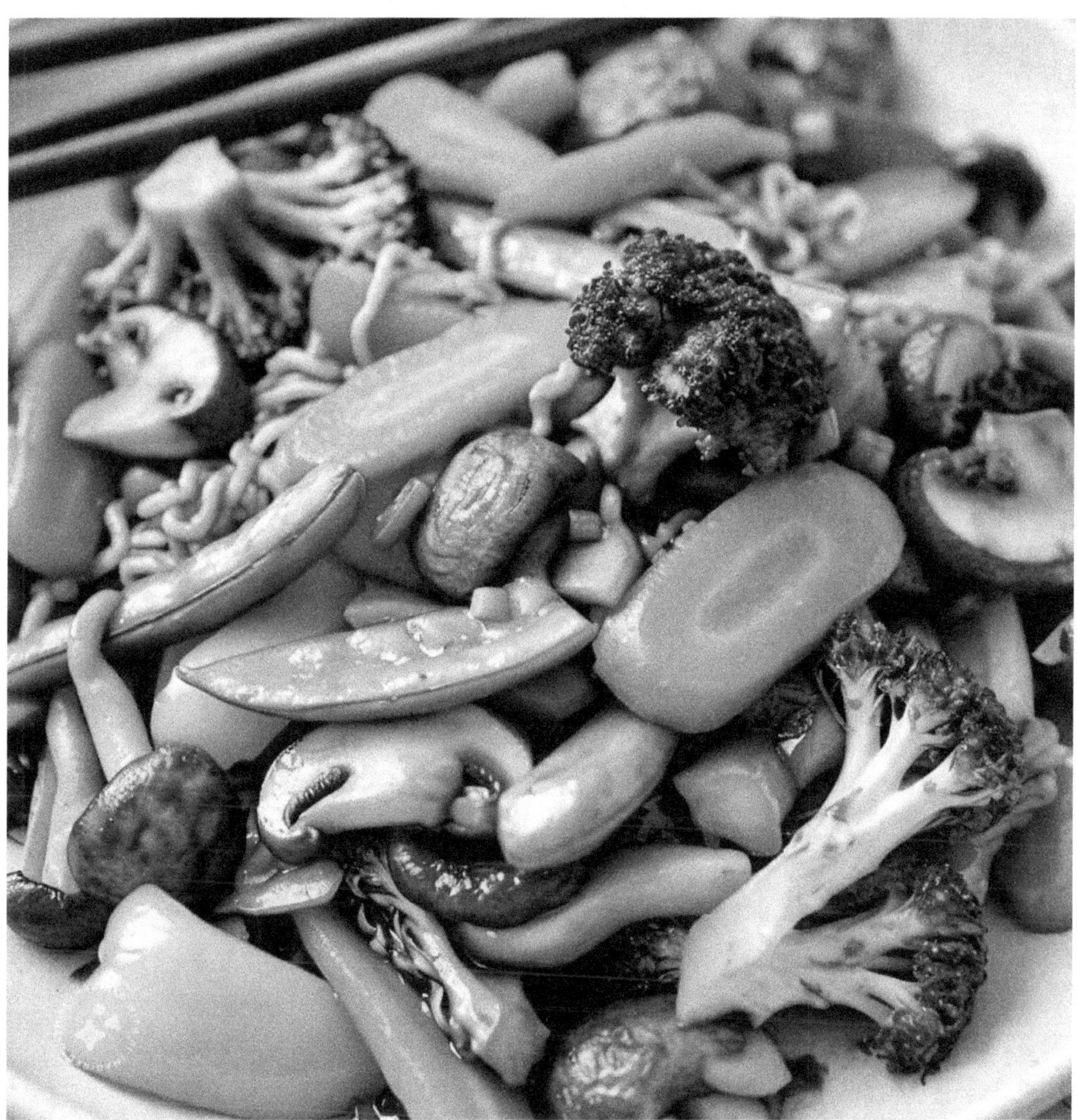

Ingredients:

- 2 tbsp vegetable oil (or sesame oil for flavor)

- 1 onion, sliced

- 2-3 garlic cloves, minced

- 1-inch piece of fresh ginger, minced

- 1 bell pepper, sliced

- 1 carrot, thinly sliced

- 1 zucchini, sliced

- 1 cup broccoli florets

- 1/2 cup snap peas

- 1 cup mushrooms, sliced

- 2-3 tbsp soy sauce (or tamari for gluten-free)

- 1 tbsp sesame oil (for flavor)

- 1 tbsp rice vinegar (optional)

- 1-2 tbsp hoisin sauce or oyster sauce (optional for extra flavor)

- 1 tsp sesame seeds (for garnish)

- Fresh cilantro or green onions (optional, for garnish)

- Cooked rice or noodles, for serving

Instructions:

1. **Prepare the Vegetables:**

   - Slice all the vegetables into bite-sized pieces. Keep the harder vegetables like carrots and broccoli separate, as they take longer to cook.

2. **Heat the Oil:**

   - Heat 2 tablespoons of vegetable oil (or sesame oil) in a large skillet or wok over medium-high heat.

3. **Sauté Aromatics:**

   - Add the minced garlic and ginger to the hot oil and sauté for 30 seconds to 1 minute until fragrant, being careful not to burn them.

4. **Stir-Fry the Vegetables:**

- Add the onions, carrots, and broccoli to the skillet and stir-fry for 3-4 minutes until they start to soften.

- Add the bell pepper, zucchini, snap peas, and mushrooms, and stir-fry for another 3-5 minutes until all the vegetables are tender-crisp.

5. **Add the Sauce:**

- Pour in the soy sauce, sesame oil, and rice vinegar (if using). Stir to coat the vegetables evenly. If you want a sweeter, richer flavor, add hoisin or oyster sauce at this point. Cook for another 2 minutes.

6. **Serve:**

- Remove from heat and garnish with sesame seeds, fresh cilantro, or green onions, if desired. Serve over steamed rice or noodles.

45. Margherita Pizza

Made with fresh tomatoes and mozzarella, this pizza provides a good blend of vitamins, healthy fats, and flavor.

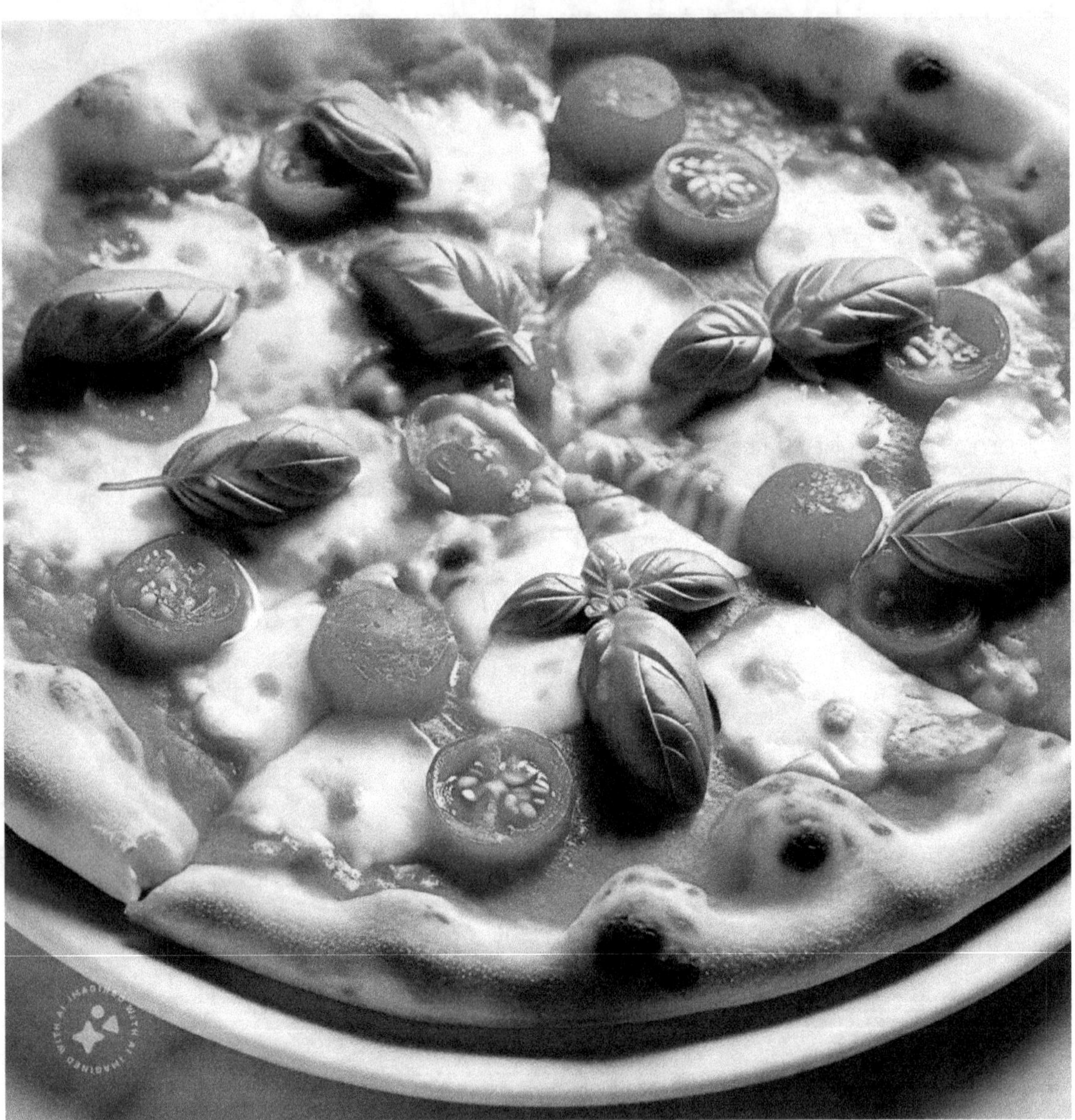

Ingredients:

For the Dough:

- 2 1/4 tsp active dry yeast (1 packet)

- 1 tsp sugar

- 3/4 cup warm water (110°F/45°C)

- 2 cups all-purpose flour

- 1 tsp salt

- 1 tbsp olive oil

For the Toppings:

- 1/2 cup pizza sauce (or crushed tomatoes seasoned with salt and pepper)

- 8 oz fresh mozzarella, sliced

- 2-3 ripe tomatoes, thinly sliced

- Fresh basil leaves

- 1-2 tbsp olive oil

- Salt and freshly ground black pepper, to taste

Instructions:

1. Prepare the Dough:

- In a small bowl, combine the warm water, yeast, and sugar. Stir and let sit for 5-10 minutes until the yeast becomes frothy.

- In a large mixing bowl, combine the flour and salt. Make a well in the center, pour in the yeast mixture and olive oil, and mix until a dough forms.

- Knead the dough on a floured surface for about 5-7 minutes until smooth and elastic.

- Place the dough in an oiled bowl, cover with a kitchen towel, and let it rise in a warm place for 1 hour, or until doubled in size.

2. Preheat the Oven:

- Preheat your oven to 475°F (245°C). If using a pizza stone, place it in the oven while it heats up.

3. **Shape the Dough:**

   - Punch down the dough and roll it out on a floured surface into a thin circle (about 10-12 inches in diameter). Transfer the dough to a pizza peel or a baking sheet lined with parchment paper if not using a pizza stone.

4. **Add the Toppings:**

   - Spread a thin layer of pizza sauce over the dough, leaving a small border for the crust.

   - Arrange the fresh mozzarella slices evenly over the sauce, followed by the tomato slices.

   - Drizzle a little olive oil over the top and season with salt and pepper.

5. **Bake the Pizza:**

   - Transfer the pizza to the oven (onto the preheated stone, if using) and bake for 10-12 minutes, or until the crust is golden and crispy, and the cheese is melted and bubbly.

6. **Add Fresh Basil:**

   - Once the pizza is out of the oven, scatter fresh basil leaves over the top. Let the pizza cool for a minute or two before slicing and serving.

46. Greek Salad

Rich in antioxidants, healthy fats, and protein from feta cheese, Greek salad is a light and refreshing lunch choice.

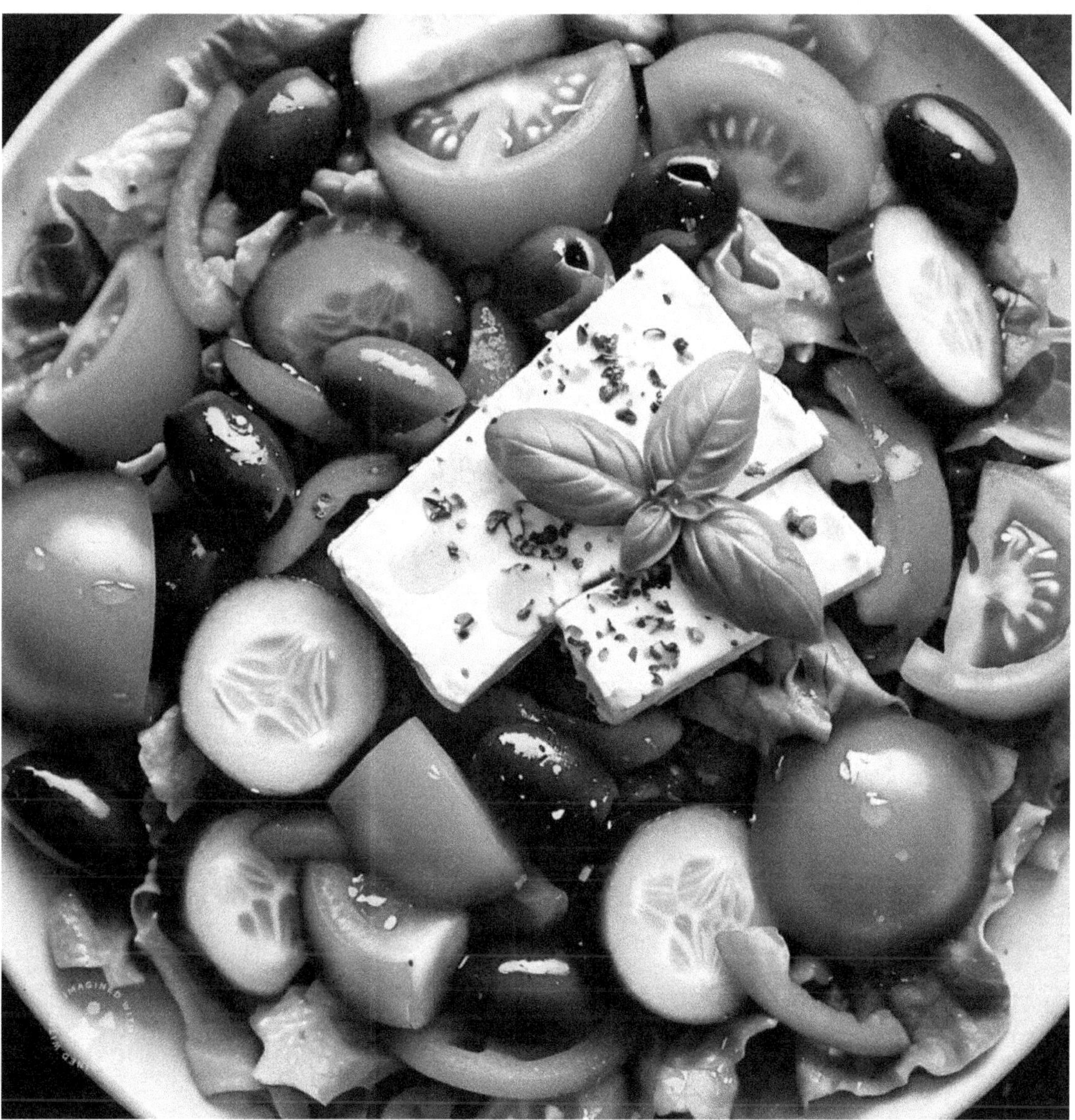

Ingredients:

- 4 ripe tomatoes, cut into wedges or large chunks

- 1 cucumber, sliced into half-moons

- 1/2 red onion, thinly sliced

- 1/2 cup Kalamata olives

- 1 green bell pepper, thinly sliced (optional)

- 8 oz feta cheese, cut into cubes or crumbled

- 2-3 tbsp extra virgin olive oil

- 1 tbsp red wine vinegar (optional)

- 1 tsp dried oregano

- Salt and freshly ground black pepper, to taste

- Fresh parsley for garnish (optional)

Instructions:

1. **Prepare the Vegetables:**

   - In a large bowl, combine the tomato wedges, cucumber slices, red onion, olives, and green bell pepper (if using).

2. **Add the Feta:**

   - Add the cubes or crumbled feta cheese to the salad. You can either mix it in gently or leave it on top as a garnish.

3. **Make the Dressing:**

   - Drizzle the extra virgin olive oil over the salad. If you like a bit of acidity, add 1 tablespoon of red wine vinegar.

   - Sprinkle with dried oregano, and season with salt and freshly ground black pepper.

4. **Toss the Salad:**

   - Toss the salad gently to combine all the ingredients and evenly distribute the dressing.

5. **Serve:**

   - Garnish with fresh parsley, if desired, and serve immediately.

47. Stuffed Grape Leaves

These leaves, a Mediterranean staple, are packed with nutrient-dense grains and herbs that aid digestion and cardiovascular health.

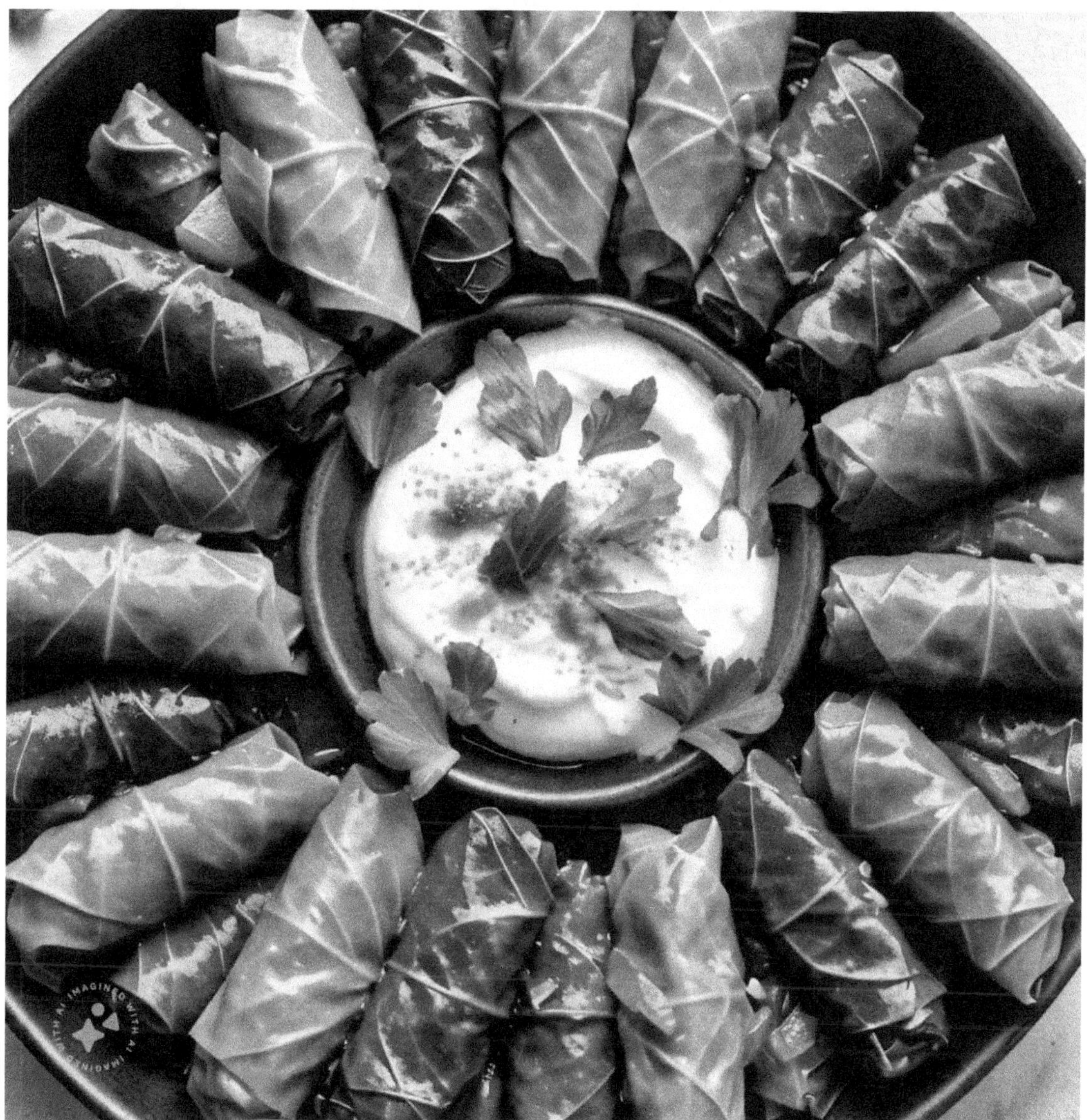

Ingredients:

- 1 jar grape leaves (about 40-50 leaves), rinsed and drained

- 1 1/2 cups short-grain rice (like Arborio)

- 1 small onion, finely chopped

- 3 cloves garlic, minced

- 1/4 cup fresh parsley, chopped

- 1/4 cup fresh dill, chopped

- 1/4 cup fresh mint, chopped

- 1/4 cup pine nuts (optional)

- 1/4 cup raisins or currants (optional)

- 1/4 cup olive oil (plus extra for drizzling)

- Juice of 2 lemons

- 1 tsp ground allspice (optional)

- Salt and pepper to taste

- 3-4 cups vegetable or chicken broth (for simmering)

Instructions:

1. **Prepare the Filling:**

   - Heat 2 tablespoons of olive oil in a skillet over medium heat. Add the chopped onion and garlic, and sauté for 3-4 minutes until softened.

   - Stir in the rice and cook for 2-3 minutes, stirring occasionally. Add the chopped parsley, dill, mint, pine nuts, and raisins (if using), and season with salt, pepper, and ground allspice. Remove from heat and let the filling cool.

2. **Prepare the Grape Leaves:**

   - Rinse the grape leaves thoroughly to remove excess brine. Pat them dry with a clean towel. Trim any tough stems from the leaves.

3. **Stuff the Grape Leaves:**

   - Place a grape leaf on a flat surface with the shiny side down and the stem end facing you. Add about 1 tablespoon of the rice filling in the center near the stem.

Fold the sides of the leaf over the filling, then roll it up tightly, like a burrito. Repeat with the remaining grape leaves and filling.

4. **Layer and Cook the Dolmas:**

- In a large pot, drizzle a little olive oil and cover the bottom with a few unused or torn grape leaves to prevent sticking.

- Arrange the stuffed grape leaves seam-side down in the pot, packing them snugly in layers.

5. **Simmer the Dolmas:**

- Pour the lemon juice and the remaining olive oil over the stuffed grape leaves. Add enough broth to the pot to cover the dolmas.

Place a heavy plate or lid over the top to keep them from unrolling while cooking.

- Bring the liquid to a simmer over low heat and cook for about 45-60 minutes, or until the rice is tender.

6. **Serve:**

- Allow the dolmas to cool to room temperature before serving. Drizzle with extra olive oil and serve with lemon wedges.

48. Tomato and Basil Bruschetta

Tomatoes contain antioxidants and vitamins, while basil has anti-inflammatory characteristics, making this a heart-healthy snack.

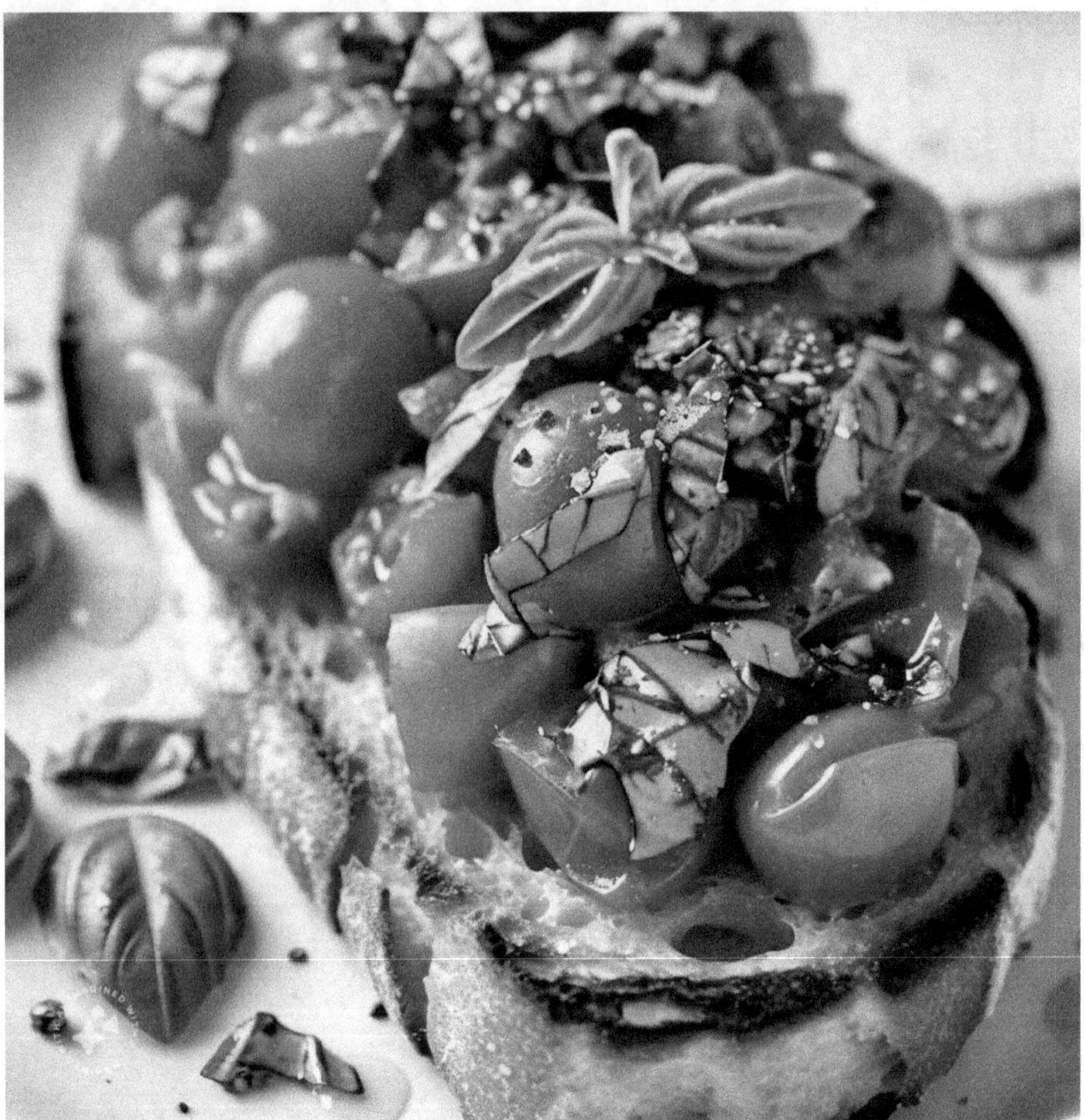

Ingredients:

- 4-6 slices of rustic or Italian bread (like ciabatta or baguette)

- 4 ripe tomatoes, diced

- 1/4 cup fresh basil leaves, chopped

- 2-3 cloves garlic, peeled and halved

- 3-4 tbsp extra virgin olive oil (plus extra for drizzling)

- 1 tbsp balsamic vinegar (optional)

- Salt and freshly ground black pepper, to taste

- Parmesan cheese or mozzarella (optional)

Instructions:

1. **Prepare the Tomato Topping:**

   - In a bowl, combine the diced tomatoes, chopped basil, 3-4 tablespoons of olive oil, and balsamic vinegar (if using). Season with salt and pepper to taste. Set aside to let the flavors meld for 10-15 minutes.

2. **Grill the Bread:**

   - Heat a grill or grill pan to medium-high heat. Lightly brush both sides of the bread slices with olive oil.

   - Grill the bread for 1-2 minutes on each side, until golden brown and crispy.

3. **Rub with Garlic:**

   - While the bread is still warm, rub one side of each slice with the cut side of the garlic cloves. This will infuse the bread with a mild garlic flavor.

4. **Assemble the Bruschetta:**

   - Spoon the tomato and basil mixture over the grilled bread slices. Drizzle with a little extra olive oil, if desired.

5. **Serve:**

   - Serve the bruschetta immediately as an appetizer or snack. You can optionally top with shavings of Parmesan cheese or slices of fresh mozzarella for an extra touch.

49. Spinach and Feta Stuffed Peppers

This low-carb, nutrient-dense meal is high in vitamins and protein from spinach and feta.

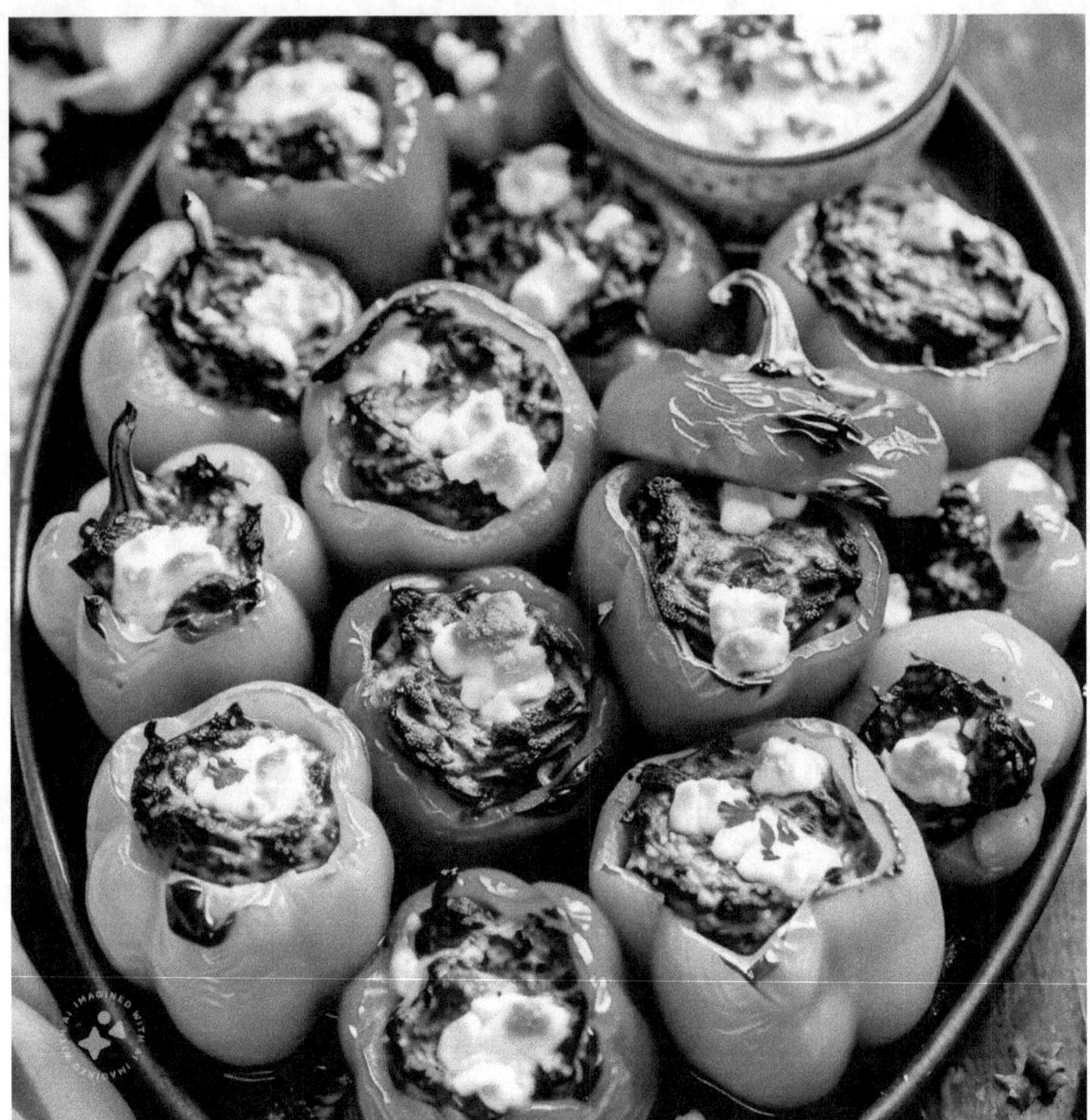

Ingredients:

- 4 large bell peppers (any color)

- 1 cup cooked quinoa

- 2 cups fresh spinach, chopped

- 1 cup feta cheese, crumbled

- 1/2 cup onion, finely chopped

- 2-3 cloves garlic, minced

- 1/4 cup sun-dried tomatoes, chopped (optional)

- 1/2 tsp dried oregano

- 1/2 tsp dried basil

- Salt and pepper, to taste

- 1 tbsp olive oil

- 1/2 cup vegetable or chicken broth (for baking)

Instructions:

1. **Preheat the Oven:**

   - Preheat your oven to 375°F (190°C).

2. **Prepare the Bell Peppers:**

   - Slice the tops off the bell peppers and remove the seeds and membranes. If needed, trim the bottom slightly so they can stand upright. Place the peppers upright in a baking dish.

3. **Sauté the Filling:**

   - In a skillet, heat the olive oil over medium heat. Add the chopped onion and sauté for 3-4 minutes until translucent. Add the minced garlic and sauté for another minute until fragrant.

   - Stir in the chopped spinach and cook until wilted, about 2-3 minutes. Remove from heat.

4. **Combine the Filling:**

   - In a large bowl, combine the cooked quinoa, sautéed spinach mixture, crumbled feta cheese, sun-dried tomatoes (if using), oregano, basil, salt, and pepper. Mix well until all ingredients are combined.

5. **Stuff the Peppers:**

   - Spoon the quinoa and spinach mixture into each bell pepper, packing it down gently until filled.

6. **Bake the Peppers:**

   - Pour the vegetable or chicken broth into the bottom of the baking dish to help steam the peppers. Cover the dish with aluminum foil.

   - Bake for 30 minutes. After 30 minutes, remove the foil and bake for an additional 10-15 minutes, or until the peppers are tender and slightly charred on top.

7. **Serve:**

   - Remove from the oven and let cool slightly before serving. Enjoy your stuffed peppers warm!

50. Roasted Cauliflower Steaks

Cauliflower is a versatile, low-carb vegetable high in fiber and vitamins that promotes weight loss and digestive health.

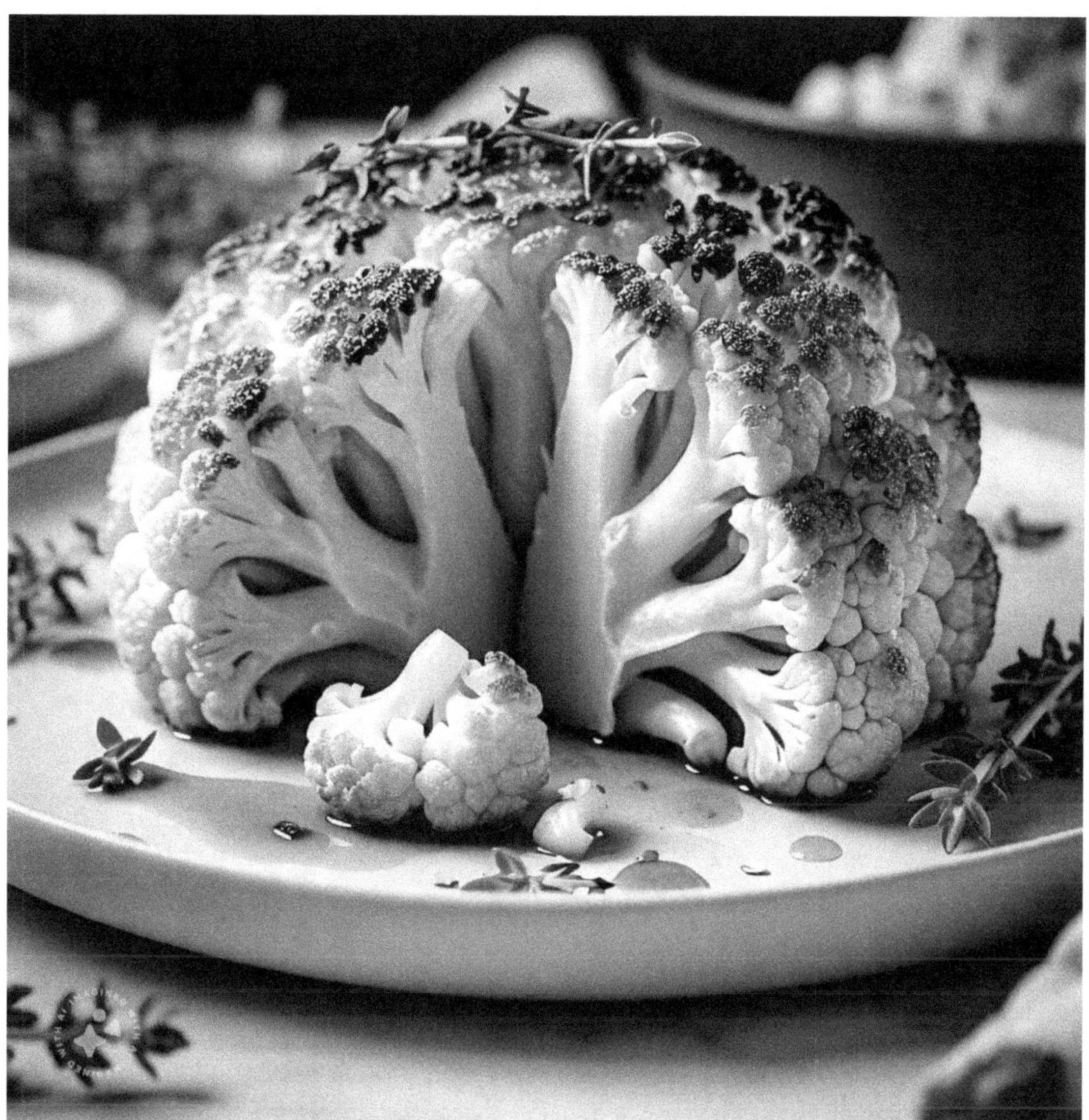

Ingredients:

- 1 large head of cauliflower

- 3-4 tbsp olive oil

- 3 cloves garlic, minced

- 1 tsp smoked paprika (or regular paprika)

- 1/2 tsp ground cumin (optional)

- Salt and freshly ground black pepper, to taste

- Fresh parsley or cilantro, for garnish (optional)

- Lemon wedges, for serving (optional)

Instructions:

1. **Preheat the Oven:**

   - Preheat your oven to 425°F (220°C). Line a baking sheet with parchment paper for easy cleanup.

2. **Prepare the Cauliflower:**

   - Remove the leaves from the cauliflower and trim the stem so that the head sits flat.

   - Using a sharp knife, slice the cauliflower into 3/4-inch to 1-inch thick steaks. You should get about 2-3 good-sized steaks from the center of the cauliflower;

   the remaining florets can be saved for another recipe or roasted alongside the steaks.

3. **Season the Cauliflower:**

   - In a small bowl, mix the olive oil, minced garlic, smoked paprika, ground cumin (if using), salt, and pepper.

   - Brush both sides of the cauliflower steaks with the olive oil mixture, ensuring they are well coated.

4. **Roast the Cauliflower:**

   - Place the cauliflower steaks on the prepared baking sheet. Roast in the preheated oven for 25-30 minutes, flipping halfway through, until they are golden brown and tender.

5. Serve:

   - Once roasted, remove the cauliflower steaks from the oven. Garnish with fresh parsley or cilantro if desired and serve with lemon wedges for squeezing over the top.

Thank you for reading this book. I hope you enjoy reading about all of these big trucks.

Please leave a review; it helps other people know they can enjoy this book.